LEFTIES

Also by Jack Fincher

Human Intelligence

LEFTIES

THE ORIGINS & CONSEQUENCES OF BEING LEFT-HANDED

**Former title
SINISTER PEOPLE**

BY JACK FINCHER

A PERIGEE BOOK

Perigee Books
are published by
G. P. Putnam's Sons
200 Madison Avenue
New York, New York 10016

Library of Congress Cataloging in Publication Data
Fincher, Jack, date.
    Lefties : the origins and consequences of being
left-handed.

    Bibliography: p.
    Includes index.
    1. Left- and right-handedness. 2. Left and right
(Psychology) 3. Brain—Localization of functions.
I. Title.
[QP385.F393   1980]   152.3'35   79-20079
ISBN 0-399-11839-X
ISBN 0-399-50460-5 Pbk.

First Perigee Printing, 1980

PRINTED IN THE UNITED STATES OF AMERICA

Second Impression

My special thanks to Dan and Carol Goltz for their editorial comments, suggestions, and fine-toothed readings. Thanks also to left-handers Patty Bock, Trevor Giles, Mark Harrison, Barbara Kaplan, Bonnie Long, Andy Mecca, Ian Murray, Mark Raus, and John Rippe for being as dependable as right-handers in returning their questionnaires. Thanks too, I guess, to Will Haymaker and Patti Sexton for just being their left-handed selves. Will returned the questionnaire too late and Patti not at all. Thanks finally to those too numerous to mention who contributed by word or deed to the genesis of this book but will, alas, find themselves not in its pages.

For My Mother,
Grace Fincher

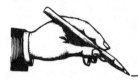

Contents

DEAR ABBY: *I am the mother of a baby who is learning to feed himself. I am almost positive that Terry is left-handed because when I put the spoon in his right hand, he transfers it to his left and proceeds eating that way.*

My husband says I should train Terry to be right-handed because everything is geared for right-handed people and the boy will be handicapped if he's left-handed. Now my husband is forcing Terry to eat with his right hand.

What do your experts say?

YOUNG MOTHER[1]

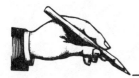# Prologue

Left-handers are one of the last surviving minorities in our society with no organization, no collective power or goals, and no real sense of common identity. The purpose of this book is to give them none of that. It is simply to examine as painlessly and informatively as possible who and what they are, and perhaps why and how they got that way.

I am, let me admit it, on balance a left-hander myself. It is nothing I planned, it just worked out that way, in spite of everything. Even this book is nothing I planned; it was suggested to me. If it seems to lack organization, a goal, collective power, and a sense of identity—well, it *is* a left-handed book, bear in mind, written more or less as a left-hander would write it. Logic is not our strong point. All-points eclecticism is.

Where logic has intruded, I have been careful to cite the source.

Since childhood, I have been enchanted by the fact and the symbolism of the right hand and the left—the one the doer, the other the dreamer. . . . Reaching for knowledge with the right hand is science. Yet to say only that much of science is to overlook one of its excitements, for the great hypotheses of science are gifts carried in the left. . . . And should we say that reaching for knowledge with the left hand is art? Again it is not enough, for as surely as the recital of a daydream differs from a well-wrought tale, there is a barrier between undisciplined fantasy and art. To climb the barrier requires a right hand adept at technique and artifice. . . . One thing has become increasingly clear in pursuing the nature of knowing. It is that the conventional [means] leaves one approach unexplored. It is an approach whose medium of exchange seems to be the metaphor paid out by the left hand. It is a way that grows happy hunches and "lucky" guesses, that is stirred into connective activity by the poet and the necromancer looking sidewise rather than directly.

—Jerome Bruner
*On Knowing: Essays
for the Left Hand*

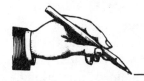

Hayfoot, Strawfoot

1

Jerome Bruner may be right, which is to say correct. Our left hand may indeed be an invaluable dreamer, a maladroit but lucky magician that finds its darkest target, as any nocturnal sharpshooter can tell you, by artfully aiming off-center.

On the other hand—witness the young mother who wrote Abigail Van Buren—I doubt society will ever see it that way. My enduring disenchantment began forty years ago, but I still remember the event as vividly as yesterday: My left hand clutching the pencil, the teacher bending over me as I mark my paper. Firmly she takes the pencil from my left hand puts it in my right, smiling encouragement. Just as firmly I return the pencil to my left and go on scribbling. She pries it from my fingers, not smiling now, puts it back in my right hand and shows me her ruler.

Not quite believing, I switch again. This time I hold on

tightly. It takes both her hands to tear the pencil loose. Now, as I watch with an interest that is not unfriendly, she squeezes the fingers of my left hand together in hers, turns it over, and—I can still feel the scalding spurt of pain and anger and surprise—beats a stinging tattoo on my palm. Fighting tears of humiliation, I put my pencil back in my right hand, where it has stayed ever since. It may well have been the first lesson I ever learned in school.

Like so many that followed, however, the lesson's rationale got lost, somewhere between the smile and the ruler. Just why left-handedness should be academically forbidden was neither evident nor ever explained. Something, we were given vaguely to understand, was wrong with it, *psychologically*. Gradually, most of us just got the idea that left-handers were intractable screwballs. And surrounded by the relentlessly right-handed equipment of the classroom, they *looked* inept, those diehard few who hadn't been saved from their manifest destiny by the high-minded interference of a dedicated first grade teacher.

It would have been inconceivable to the rest of us, those who meekly switched rather than fight, that the school might have been tinkering with the fundamental organization of our brains, the teacher innocently tampering not only with our innate ability to master language, but with the basic thrust of our thinking itself. And all because of a neurological doctrine, one now mercifully outmoded and unheeded in its severest strictures, that had the effect of making left-handedness in the classroom a social gaffe only one step up from self-abuse in the boys' room.

Parenthetically, I am indebted to my local barbershop and *True* magazine for this fascinating bit of intelligence: The fourth century B.C. poet Martial traced the common Roman expression for masturbation, *left-handed whore,* to just such a manual propensity when the ancient ladies of the evening were not around. The social significance of this distinction I am tempted to leave to the scholar. But no, more of it later.

More will be made later, too, of the arcane neurology that held sway in the American schools of my day. It may have to it, sad to say, more than a hard grain of important scientific truth—a truth that still compels some pediatricians to advise young mothers of budding left-handers to nudge the feeding dish to the right, in hopes of cutting off nature at the pass.

But what about those of us who were coerced into changing hands by more punitive action? Were we injured? Yes, modern psychology tells us, some of us were. Rarely, however, was the trauma more manifestly serious than early reading and writing problems, clumsiness, or a bad case of stuttering. *Manifestly,* it should be added, is the operative word. Who knows how many potential necromancers and poets were inadvertently detoured for a lifetime into creative cul-de-sacs? The same minor maladies that arose from such a forced switch were attributed, curiously enough, by the early neurology to unreconstructed use of the left hand. We were damned if we did and damned if we didn't.

Looking back at my own indoctrination into a dominantly right-handed world, was I permanently, devastatingly, secretly damaged? I think—at least I hope—not. As a practicing left-hander I simply and silently went underground. Or, in the negative sense of today's vernacular, into the closet. I learned to write and sharpen pencils with my right hand passably, and to draw with real skill. My transformation, though, was not without a subtle slippage in spatial orientation. Handedness, we are beginning to suspect, may be more a matter of *sidedness*—of hand, foot, eye, *and* body,

19

both inside and out, though much of the evidence remains murky.

As a rule, right-handers draw figures facing left, while left-handers do just the opposite. And I? In grade school I was once mortified, and my classmates were sent into gales of giggles, to discover that I had lost my sense of direction in midstroke and had rendered the udder of an artfully crafted cow under the *front* legs instead of the back.

In time even that sort of lateral confusion passed. Cutting figures out of construction paper, however, remained forever beyond me. So do all scissor works to this day, requiring as they do mastery of one among the countless workaday implements engineered, until recently, only for the right-handed majority: handles, screws, gearshifts, watch stems, playing cards, ice cream scoops, wrenches, rulers, phone booths, gravy boats, power saws, can openers, voting machines, vegetable peelers, slot machines, corkscrews, violins, guitars, fishing reels, bowling balls, soup ladles, pencil sharpeners, saxophones, and banjos, to name but a few.

As it was, left to my own devices at home (by two right-handed parents) and on the playground, I continued all but unfailingly, wherever practical, to increase my repertory of left-handed skills. In junior high, for example, I became left-handed marbles champ, as opposed to right-handed marbles champ. Such distinctions, as you might expect, were positively Olympian in their purity, foreshadowing those more serious in the game of life to come.

To kicking and throwing from the left, I early on added tennis and, much later, bowling. Thanks to a hand-me-down set of clubs—whose heads, like most of those throughout Western history, were dead set against my maverick predilection—I learned to golf, if wretchedly, from the right. After a successful stint of switch-hitting in softball, I decided I should bat right (like a lot of ostracized left-handers, as it happens) which may explain why I never again hit as much as my weight. Finally, bowing to social pressure, first at college, then abroad, I taught myself to change hands at the dinner table as needed. I am as adept— some would insist as maladept—with one as with the other, though I originally ate with my left and now, out of habit, prefer my right.

For that matter, after a lifetime of conditioning, I, like most left-handers, can get through the day in a world I never made without once being self-conscious about my impediment, much less demonstrating it. (My wife confesses a chronic unease at what she terms my "awkwardness" in the kitchen. But I console myself with the fact that my province is the typewriter, the one machine whose operation favors the left hand.)

From all this I have emerged with nothing more disabling than the mildest identity crisis. When asked, on those rare occasions where it seems somehow to matter, whether I am right-handed or left-handed, I never know what to say but stand, metaphorically, in the open closet doorway, smiling nervously and rubbing my guilty hands together like Pilate. If asked to take a stand, I am smitten with indecision. To cite one of the more inflammatory examples, the National League for Lefthanders—all 123 men and women strong— has been moved to suggest such militant stratagems of social protest to the rightful status quo as offering your left hand to shake, or putting stamps on the left side of letters to avoid cancellation (as if the Post Office didn't have its hands full already).

The executive director of the National League for Left-handers—an unemployed young advertising copywriter and left-handed guitar player named Robert Geden—wrote me outlining his organization's ambitious plans to form chapters, hold a national convention, lean on stores and companies to make and sell more left-handed products, pressure schools to increase left-handed facilities, and lobby government to get a fair statistical shake from the census. I sent him $5 for a silent, inactive membership, and Geden seemed glad to get it. "One thing I've discovered," he wrote back. "Too many people are apathetic, no matter how little the cost of involvement. Is it because we're supposed to be more independent-minded, or just too distinterested, or . . . ?"[1]

I sympathize, Bob. The League would find here no revolutionary firebrand seeking civil redress, just another dues-paying member of the establishment who wishes devoutly to remain uncommitted. Not for me anything like the Japan Left-handers League, which boasts 1,500 of that nation's five million left-handers and a psychiatrist founder who is now writing his second book on the subject. On the issue I am ever the muddled respondent, never the eloquent petitioner fellow left-hander Benjamin Franklin was when he penned the following:

There are twin sisters of us; and the eyes of man do not more resemble, nor are capable of being on better terms with each other than my sister and myself, were it not for the partiality of our parents, who made the most injurious distinction between us.

From my infancy I have been led to consider my sister as a being of a more educated rank. I was suffered to grow up without the least instruction, while nothing was spared in her education. She had masters to teach her writing, drawing, music and other accomplishments, but if by chance I touched a pencil, a pen or a needle I was bitterly rebuked; and more than once I have been beaten for being awkward, and wanting a graceful manner. . . .

Your obedient servant,
THE LEFT HAND[2]

Such poignant despair, I gather from the dearth of it around me, is largely at an end. In the more enlightened schools of today, children are allowed, if not encouraged, to use the hand of their choice, provided they do so with a powerful determination and don't shilly-shally around, employing first one, then the other. Knowing their own minds, educators now declare, is what is vital for developing youngsters. That may be another way of saying that if you don't make up your own mind, the school, suitably guided by expert psychological counseling, will do it for you—for your own good, of course. But ever so gently. Rulers are out, we hear. Friendly persuasion, the drip-drip-drip of repeated smiling reminders, is in.

A parallel easing of tensions, a concomitant slackening of totalitarian attitudes toward the left hand, can be seen in society at large, I suppose. The celebrated (and overrated) Italian criminologist of the last century Cesare Lombroso, who conceived the low-forehead, close-set-beady-eye stereotype of the congenital wrongdoer, once called left-handedness "a stigma of degeneration."[3] He was only echoing the overwhelming bias of half the globe—one built up across a millennium of religious, philosophical, mystical, and psychiatric sensibility, prejudicial and unfounded though that may yet prove. As it happens, left-handedness is now even tolerated at the dinner table—or at least ignored by the guests, while the thoughtful hostess takes care to seat its possessor in an end chair, where the rhythmic

23

steam-shovel swoops of his offending elbow dig the darkling air and not his dinner partner's ribcage.

The right-minded majority, in short, appears ready to make its necessary peace with yet another implacably troublesome minority. And just in time, too, since left-handers are surviving our schools' new permissiveness at such a brisk clip that the popularly accepted nine-to-one ratio between preferred hands has become just one more iffy paradigm wafting on the winds of change. The number of left-hand writers, in fact, has all but *doubled* in the last decade.

All in all, just how many left-handers are there? The question cannot be answered because it has not been properly asked. But one thing is certain. There may be many more sinister (from the Latin for left) skeletons in the *Homo sapiens* closet than we ever suspected. Perhaps you, Dear Reader, wholly unknowing, are among them.

In any event, the left-hander today can even buy some fifty or so items designed expressly for his needs, including his own reversely-strung guitar, moustache mug, can-opener (a luxury version of the standard Danish Army issue) and—my old first grade teacher take note—a ruler with the numbers running right to left.

And why not? A Connecticut mail order firm sees a hefty market of twenty million customers in this country—even as a toolmaker in Milan, Italy, hit the mercantile jackpot with—brace yourself, all your practical jokers—a left-handed monkey wrench. There are even shops in New York, London, and Boston where the left-hander can freely browse, in a counter-clockwise direction, of course (a heretical notion in most stores), buy an ambidextrous tea-pot with a double spout made by the owner's left-handed Aunt Pearl, pick up copies of Prokofiev's Concerto No. 4 for the Left Hand and Ravel's Concerto in D Major for the Left Hand for Piano and Orchestra, put on a "Kiss Me, I'm

Left-Handed" button, shake hands somberly with a left-handed dog.

Something called The Association for the Protection of the Rights of Left-Handers now exists, we are further told, and campaigns for the allowable use of the left hand in taking oaths and saluting—something an executive I know did in the army with distressing regularity. "They damned near drummed me out," he remembers. Dentists can get left-handed equipment, moreover, and some banks have reportedly started issuing checkbooks with stubs on the right side.

Even so, the left-hander cannot be blamed for wondering if his cause, like so many others, hasn't been slyly preempted. (Assuming he has a cause. It is all but hidden, even to himself.) The psychic scar tissue of the outcast is tough, to be sure. But the wound, however complete the healing, goes deep and tends to ache whenever the emotional climate changes. And just look at that place setting. You can't help noticing your fork is still laid out on the same side as everybody else's. For some things don't change. As a gifted athlete I know laments, "It's always been a drag playing baseball and loving the positions of shortstop and catcher—always from a left-handed distance."

I'm sure his sentiments would be echoed in essence by a concert violinist, if I knew one. Beneath its newly mannered surface, the aging cold war continues.

But enough of such maunderings. Speaking rhetorically on behalf of society, who *are* these guys, anyway? (Most of them are male.) Where and what on earth do they spring from, and why? What, if anything, is the significance of their phenomenon to themselves and the rest of us? And what, to put a grand sound to it, is the meaning of their renegade existence for our tumultuous times?

Bruner's metaphor may be accurate. Perhaps, in the

brainiest sense, it may even be more accurate than he imagines. But what about his—and other—facts?

True enough, the left-handed, like the poor, have always been with us. It is perfectly true, too, that a statistically disproportionate number of them have been alcoholics, bed wetters, poor achievers, slow learners, and chronic misfits; figuratively speaking, square pegs the culture has pushed into round holes. And—criminologists take note—a couple of them turned out to be two of our most infamous antisocials: Jack the Ripper and the Boston Strangler.

But an impressive host of others have, by their feats and natures, both illumined the history of the world and brightened the corners where we briefly are. What better time, and way, to salute their persistence, pluck, and enterprise than by a roll call of those known to be from their broad and illustrious company of irregulars down through the ages?

So, left-handers, front and center.

Stepping perversely off on your right foot, of course. That was the practice of Western military man until King Frederick William I of Prussia in the eighteenth century decided something drastic was needed to instill the kind of discipline that wins wars. What better tactic than to make recruits put not their best foot forward, but, in the eyes of the Western world, their worst?

(The Prussian style swiftly spread, giving rise in one European country to the legend that its soldiers were so dense they could only march if hay were tied to one foot, straw to the other, and the command given, "Hayfoot, strawfoot!")

And here they come! (Hayfoot, strawfoot.)

Alexander the Great, Judy Garland, Gerald Ford, Marilyn Monroe, Leonardo da Vinci, F. Lee Bailey, Betty Grable, Jim Bishop, Ringo Starr, Ronald Reagan, Herschel Bernardi, Casey Stengel, Rock Hudson, Robert Blake, Ben

Franklin, Harpo Marx, James A. Garfield, Vikki Carr, Carol Burnett, Hans Holbein, Lenny Bruce, Ronald Searle, Rudy Vallee, Bill Mauldin, Tiny Tim, Raphael, Joey Heatherton, Paul McCartney, Rod Laver, Danny Kaye, Robert Redford, King George VI, Jimi Hendrix, Hope Lange, Michael Landon, Chuck Connors, Jim Hutton, Cleavon Little, Babe Ruth, Charlie Chaplin, Don Rickles, Uri Geller, Robert Morse, Euell Gibbons, Terry Thomas, Mark Spitz, Ryan O'Neal, Rod Steiger, Cole Porter, James Whitmore, Rip Torn, Milton Caniff, Allen Funt, Paul Williams, Cloris Leachman, Pablo Picasso, Keenan Wynn, Nelson Rockefeller, Michelangelo (maybe), Eva Marie Saint, Charlemagne, Kim Novak, Ken Stabler, Peter Fonda, Lou Gehrig, Rex Harrison, Jimmy Connors, Dick Van Dyke, Arnold Palmer, Hans Conreid, Ted Williams, Ann Meara, Stan Musial, Dick Smothers, Lord Nelson, Richard Dreyfuss, McGeorge Bundy, Jack Carter, James L. Corbett, Peggy Cass, Clarence Darrow, Marie Dionne, Marty Engles, Queen Mother Elizabeth, Henry Ford Jr., Lefty Gomez, Lefty Grove, George Gobel, Lou Harris, Huntington Hartford, Ben Hogan, Herbert Hoover, Jim Lucas, Allen Ludden, Rube Marquard, Robert S. McNamara, Marcel Marceau, Edward R. Murrow, Anthony Newley, Robert Preston, Jean Seberg, Warren Spahn, Emperor Tiberius, Henry Wallace, Queen Victoria, Paul Klee, Caroline Kennedy, and Lewis Carroll, who stuttered.

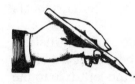# Is God Right-Handed?

2

Was Adam left-handed? Better yet, was Eve? When the metaphorical Mother of Us All reached out for the forbidden fruit, committing the original sin that led to our everlasting banishment from Paradise, which hand did she use?

On this point Genesis is mute—strangely so, as we shall see. And judging from a spot check of religious art down through the ages, the question, if ever asked, remains unanswered. Four artists, including Michelangelo, depict Eve holding or taking the apple with her left hand. Four others, among them the fourteenth century Flemish master Jan van Eyck, picture just the opposite.

The issue, of course, could be hopelessly confounded by the built-in bias of the artist. Left-handers, remember, tend to face their figures to the right of the canvas. Such a preference could affect not only composition. Indirectly, in the absence of the definitive Word, it could influence theological interpretation. What, therefore, are we to make of the contribution of Michelangelo, whose handedness is a matter of some dispute? Some say he was right-handed, some left-, and some both. "During all the years I was researching and writing my book on Michelangelo I always assumed that he was right-handed," says Irving Stone, author of *The Agony and the Ecstasy.* He adds, tellingly, "Perhaps that is because I am."

Without ever getting into the handedness of the artists, it should be enough to note that, altogether, three on either side of the sample faced their figures to the left, two to the right, and three muddled matters all the more by facing them straight ahead. The eight faces of Eve, in short, are no help whatever.

For that matter, although Christ and God are always drawn bestowing blessings with the right hand, and the Devil exercising guile or hurling curses with the left, scholar Richard Uhrbrock reports a curious fact. He found a marked tendency in classical renderings of the Madonna and child for Mary to be holding Jesus not on her right but on her left. No spot-checker, Uhrbrock stared himself bleary-eyed at over a thousand paintings, drawings, and statues. What possible explanation could there be?

Well, maybe it simply "looked right," Uhrbrock offers with unconscious double entendre, because in an unrelated study of right-handed mothers in real life, eight out of ten held their child on the left, just like the Virgin Mary. Perhaps that, he concedes, was to free their right hand for other, better things.

Then again, as the original research speculates, it might be an unconscious attempt by the mother to simulate as strongly as possible the reassuring impact of her heartbeat

30

experienced by the infant before birth. That soothingly intimate thump-thump is stronger on the mother's left, and when varied in volume experimentally, it has been shown to affect an infant's crying, sleeping, and weight gain.

For some reason, Uhrbrock in his study of religious art ignores the more obvious explanation: Putting the Christ child on Mary's left puts Him on the viewer's—and the art work's—*right,* clearly the place of honor.

Admittedly, the entire argument would smack of angels and pinheads were it not for one unshakable fact: The Bible, and with it the full weight of both orthodox Judaism and Christianity, overwhelmingly favors one hand at the expense of the other. Predictably, when all the moral goodies are passed out, the scriptures come down *right*eously hard on one side, while the other, when not denigrated, is—what else?—*left* out. Both the Old and New Testament refer repeatedly to the grace and power residing in, on, or at "the right hand of God" and His only begotten son. For His part, in the sermon on the mount, Christ cryptically counsels His followers in doing charity to "let not thy left hand know what thy right hand doeth."[1]

Variations are most numerous, however—and ominously prejudicial—on the theme expressed by Jesus in the Last Judgment, according to Matthew:

> And before Him shall be gathered all nations; and He shall separate them one from another, as the shepherd dividith his sheep from the goats: And He shall set the sheep on His right hand, but the goats on the left. Then shall the King say unto them on His right hand, 'Come, ye blessed of my Father, inherit the kingdom prepared for you from the foundation of the world. . . .' Then shall He say unto them on the left hand, 'Depart from me, ye cursed, into everlasting fire, prepared for the devil and his angels. . . .'[2]

31

Bad luck, surely. But the Old Testament does little better. For example, God tells Jonah that Nineveh, that wicked city, contains people so sinful they "cannot discern between their right hand and their left hand,"[3] presumably, we are left to infer, between good and bad.

Only once, in fact, does the left-hander have anything like his just innings, and this in a warlike, ultimately disastrous context. Among 26,000 Benjamites (curiously, from "Ben Yamin," meaning literally "Son of the Right Hand"[4]), we are told in Judges, were

seven hundred chosen men lefthanded; every one could sling stones at an hair breadth, and not miss.[5]

For that reason, perhaps, it took several fierce battles and a brisk series of pep talks from the Lord before the Children of Israel put the tribe of Benjamin to bloody flight. Scripturally speaking, the left-hander's lot has gone steadily downhill ever since, in both words and pictures. Indeed, according to Jane Dillenberger, an authority on Biblical art at the Graduate Theological Seminary in Berkeley, the overweening right-handedness of its symbolism is as near to an absolute as anything in the Judeo-Christian tradition.

But why?

Dillenberger and the Judeo-Christian tradition are at a scholarly loss to answer. When pressed, Dillenberger replies, in effect, that it just—*is*, that's all. Church ritual certainly bears her out. The offering and taking of the Communion wafer of bread and chalice of wine, the movements of priest and communicant, the Sign of the Cross and the Benediction—all are right in character. To do otherwise is blasphemy.

At that, both Judaism and Christianity merely reflect the

prevailing sentiments of Western civilization. Ancient Athens professed to see any fall from symmetry as just another example of man's ungodly imperfection. Aristophanes declared that man had been created round, with his moon face to heaven and his great, single, spherical butt as invincibly grounded in gravity as one of those toy clowns you knock over only to have it bounce cheerily upright again. To these perfect specimens centered in utmost spherical serenity, wrote Aristophanes, there was no front or back, no left or right, no "wrong" or "right" side.

Alas, they grew so arrogant and haughty that Zeus in his anger split them into halves and tossed these to Apollo, who turned the new-made face and genitals of each raw hemisphere forward so they might better heed their Maker's warning:

"If they continue impertinent, I shall split them once more and they will hop along on one leg."[6]

Once man's divine symmetry was broken, however, the classical Greeks for all their aesthetic sophistication proved no more able to resist a rightful bias than anyone else. Jamblichus, in his *Life of Pythagoras,* disclosed that the master recommended his disciples "enter holy places by the right, which is . . . divine, and leave them by the left, the symbol of . . . dissolution."[7] That the Pythagoreans complied with a vengeance would later be confirmed by Aristotle, who observed that they "call good what is on the right, above and in front, and bad what is on the left, below and behind."[8] Indeed, Plutarch reports, in crossing their legs they took care never to put their left on top of their right. Parmenides went even further. He extended that injunction into the very womb itself. The origin of the sexes, he decreed, depended upon the position of the fetus in the mother. Boys were on one side, girls on the other, and it doesn't take a card-carrying feminist to guess which was which.

As one Athenian might have remarked to another at the pinnacle of such a discourse, What does Plato say? The man to whose thinking the rest of Western philosophy has been called "a series of footnotes"[9] was plainly of two warring minds. On the one hand he hailed the Pythagorean viewpont as expressing the essential harmonies that govern the universe. In the myth of Er the Pamphylian, for example, Plato speaks in by-now-familiar tones of how the soul, when it leaves the body, journeys until it reaches a wondrous place where

> the judges sit between two openings; when they have pronounced their sentences, they order the just to take the right-hand road which leads to Heaven, after having attached to them, in front, a decree setting forth their judgment; but they order criminals to take the left-hand path leading downwards, they also carrying, but attached behind, a document on which is written all their deeds.[10]

Since, so far as we know, Jesus could neither read nor write Greek, such moral long-division must have been a myth of remarkable popularity and staying power.

This pin-the-tail-on-the-donkey polemic, on the other hand, is strangely at variance with the practical Plato, who was quite a hard-headed social critic for his times. Foreshadowing the cultural observations of Plutarch's *Moralia* almost five centuries later, Plato takes a long and critical look at the forces of Greek conformity and laments them through his Athenian stranger in *The Laws:*

> *The Athenian:* . . . There is a prejudice about which almost no one can do anything.

34

Cleinias: What prejudice?

The Athenian: That of believing that in all our actions there is a natural difference between right and left [hands. . . .] The stupidity of nurses and mothers has made us all one-armed. . . . Indeed, the natural aptitude of the two arms is the same, and it is ourselves who have made them unequal and who do not use them as we should.[11]

Plato's ambivalence is curiously politic. His conclusion—we are all guilty, but those stupid women did it—smacks of Richard Nixon on Watergate: As a man Plato accepts his share of responsibility; as a philosopher he refuses to be blamed.

The Greeks, nonetheless, in both myth and culture, continued faithfully and forcefully to relay the tradition their leading thinker had dismissed as groundless. So, too, did the later Christians, who embraced as gospel the legend that saints in their cradle were so pious they refused to suck from the left breast of their mother.

No people, however, were more zealous in promoting the right than the Romans. With an empire to propagate its superiority, they adopted the right-hand handshake, the Fascist salute, and—momentously—a left-to-right alphabet to articulate such insidious and polarizing concepts as *dexter* for right (as in dextrous: skillful, artful, clever) and *sinister* for left (as in baleful, malign, dire.) They all but went the Pythagoreans one better. Entering a friend's home, they were careful always to put their right foot forward. To the rightful Roman mind, even sneezing, depending on which way you turned your head, was an augury of fortune, good or bad. Originally, left was the lucky side. But the practice of augury soon fell into disrepute as the shady domain of charlatans. When it was once again welcomed back into re-

35

spectable society, wouldn't you know it, the lucky side had become the right.

Christianity, in contrast, was a rock of righteous resolve. Today, when we spill salt, most of us absently pick up some of it in our right hand and toss it over our left shoulder. We little know or care that such a gesture originated when Judas was depicted as having spilled the salt in da Vinci's *The Last Supper*. We are acting, legend has it, to propitiate the Devil, who of course lurks in that God-forsaken vicinity behind our left shoulder.

Feudalism further fostered our rightward trend in the Middle Ages, when the king's favorite sat on his right hand (thus becoming his "right-hand man"), while the *bar sinister* was bestowed by a grudging heraldry on the bastard son, whose claim to the throne was regarded as illegitimate, unlucky, and evil. The same practice was extended to the physical layout of the prerevolutionary French National Assembly, giving us a set of political labels—and some would say attitudes—that exist to this day. The nobles were the governments' "right" wing, the then-upstart capitalists, of all people, its "left" wing.

Although precise data are sketchy, simple logic suggests that the left-hander's lot must have taken a quantum jump for the worse with the Industrial Revolution. Machine-made tools meant that he had better learn to make his maladroit (not dextrous; hence, not *right*, as opposed to *adroit*, or dextrous) best of a bad arrangement. Who could afford to mass-produce anything for the one man in many?

Truth to tell, when the Ambidexteral Cultural Society was established in England at the turn of this century on the laudable proposition that everyone should learn to use *either* hand equally, industry did not rise up and strike a blow for equity by differentiating its manufacturing dies.

The sanctity of right-handed tools was implicit. For that matter, our enduring bias stood nakedly revealed in the very word itself. Ambidextrous actually means "right-handed on both sides." It also means "hypocritical" or "deceptive"—which, come to think of it, is a pretty accurate description of the whole sorry affair.

In fact, language has always betrayed our ingrained prejudice. Despite the more enlightened early Greeks, who in a presumably weak moment gave their word for left, *aristera*, to the aristocrats ("those best qualified to govern"), the left-hander has stayed linguistically on the outs with Western civilization from the beginning.

Left, in a word, is almost universally bad. *Mancino* means "deceitful" in Italian; *linkisch* " awkward" in German; *na levo* "sneaky" in Russian. In Spanish *zurdo* also means "malicious," and *no ser zurdo*, "to be not left-handed," in addition means "to be very clever." *Cack-handed*, from the colloquial English word *cack* for excrement (the French *caca*), is British slang for sinistral, while the *macho* Australians let you know what they think of such an infirmity by calling the left-handed a *molly-dooker* or "woman-handed."

The English word *left*, as a matter of fact, has no more respectable antecedents. It comes from the Anglo-Saxon *lyft*, an offshoot of the Old Dutch, meaning "weak" or "broken." *Riht*, in contrast, is Anglo-Saxon for straight, erect, or just. In modern usage, moreover, the French word for left, *gauche* (originally: "bent" or "askew") is applied to those social misfits who make a habit of putting their foot in their mouth. Conversely, the French word for right, *droit*, also means "correct" and "law." We all know what not being "on the side of law" signifies. It signifies, naturally, not going "straight"—which the pedantic French, to put an

37

even finer point on it, overkill with the expression *tout droit:* "wholly, entirely right." A Gallic cousin, no doubt, to the English word *upright.*

No wonder, then, that a left-handed oath is never to be trusted, that the evil eye is on the left, that in witchcraft evil spells are cast by laying on the left hand, that in the marriage ceremony right hands are joined, but the wedding ring is put on the third finger of the left hand—the "charm finger" in superstition—to ward off black magic with the power thought to reside in the precious metal.

Small wonder, too, that free men are born with a birthright, stand up for their rights when they are wronged, and prize the Bill of Rights as one of their most cherished possessions. Right? *Right on!*

Smaller wonder still that psychiatry, the secular faith of modern man, has joined religion in looking askance at the sinistral. How could it do otherwise when the very unconscious is infected with such distinctions? In his wry and amusing paper, "Why Did They Sit on the King's Right?" William Domhoff reports that the case histories of psychiatric patients are riddled with left-right imagery:

> One American psychoanalyst described a patient's dream in which writing with the left hand meant doing things the wrong way. . . . In interpreting a dream in which a car hit an obstruction and swerved to the left, still another psychoanalyst explained that "the left side of this patient, as is common, represented his weaker, and thus feminine side."[12]

Most fascinating to Domhoff was a young female patient who

> used to see herself in a mental picture as two persons, a right and a left Rose, and told me exactly what each of them

was doing, and saying. . . . It appeared that the right one was her good self, while the left was a delinquent and utterly wicked child who could not be tolerated by the better self.[13]

Such a split has far-reaching implications. "Among other things," writes one of Jung's disciples, " 'right' often means, psychologically, the side of conscious, of adaptation, of being 'right,' while 'left' signifies the sphere of unadapted, unconscious reactions."[14]

As we shall see when we examine the basic organization of our brains, he, like Bruner, may have been even righter than he knew.

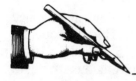

Sinister Savages

3

But getting back to the central question, why should this enduring disparity in human handedness be? For what reason has history so preferred our right and singled out our left for such unrelenting infamy? If, as Plato concluded, there is nothing natural about it, how are we to explain such a persisting and curious phenomenon?

The jury is still out, but let's take a long and searching look at human mentality itself for possible clues to the eventual verdict. Take Plato, for instance. Putting aside for the moment the practical Plato, let us address our inquiry to the mythic, the religious, the philosophic side of this most profound thinker. What does he find so universal, so essential, so harmonious, and therefore so clearly satisfying about the either/or dichotomy inherent in opposing hands?

Obviously the answer, if there is one, must lie in the symmetrical nature of such sidedness, in the balance it achieves by its very polarity. Other spatial opposites abound in life, of course, and are just as commonly freighted with all the metaphysical baggage they can carry—to name but a few: up and down (Heaven and Hell), back and front (past and future), inner and outer (subjective and objective reality).

More to the point are the observations of the French sociologist Robert Hertz, whose minor classic of meticulous investigation, *The Pre-Eminence of The Right Hand,* has not been materially diminished by the passing of sixty-five years. Indeed, that may explain why an English language version was brought out as late as 1960. Hertz eloquently argues that human hands are the inevitable symbols of all the fundamental dualisms underlying religious thought: good and evil, sacred and profane, the divine and the demoniac. This is because, as one Oxford commentator on his work phrased it, "the duality in the universe of ideas must be centered in man who is the center of them."[1]

Or as Hertz himself said, "How could man's body, the microcosm, escape the law of polarity which governs everything?"[2] Seen that way, Christ's injunction to let not the left hand know what the right hand does makes tidy sense, obeying as it does "this law of the incompatibility of opposites."[3]

In support of his thesis, Hertz musters a formidable body of anthropoligical evidence. His many proofs range from the moral distinctions the primitive Maori culture of the South Pacific makes between the male side of all things (*virile, creative, alive, strong, sacred*) and the female (its antithesis), to North American Indian sign language, in which the right hand, when elevated, connotes such bracing positives as *self, high estate, bravery,* and *power,* but when turned to the left and lowered beneath its sinister opposite, stands for the negativity of death, destruction, and burial.

Like Plato, Hertz holds no brief for the inherent superi-

42

ority of either hand. But as his research makes amply evident, around the globe the two sides of man are almost uniformly regarded like the politicized classes of George Orwell's *Animal Farm:* Both are equal, but one is more equal than the other.

"The left," Hertz reports of its usual treatment, "is the hand of perjury, treachery and fraud." In the rites of worship across eastern Russia, "the gods are on our right, so we turn towards the right to pray. A holy place must be entered right foot first. Sacred offerings are presented to the gods with the right hand."[4] Similarly, in rituals of consecration far removed in time, place, and deity, societies as diverse as the Hindus and Celts mutually "go three times round a person or object, from left to right."[5] Sinners, moreover, notes Hertz, are traditionally expelled from the Catholic church through the left door.

Nor do spiritual prohibitions against the sinister stop there. On the contrary, "the dominion of religious concepts is so powerful that it makes itself felt in the dining room, the kitchen, and even in those places haunted by demons and which we dare not name."[6] Even the simple act of eating with the right hand, Hertz believes, springs from the fact that many primitive peoples, when in an "impure" state—mourning, for instance—may not use their hands for eating. If they did, they would "swallow their own death."[7] When initiated into the solemn craft of weaving by their priest, he found, Maori women must take care to weave the ceremonial thread from left to right with their right hand— or suffer certain profanation and death, too. Among the tribes of Africa's lower Niger river, women also are forbidden to use their left hand when cooking, for fear of poisonous sorcery.

Indeed, writes Hertz:

43

Among the Maori the expression *tama tane,* "male side," designates . . . men's virility, descent in the paternal line . . . creative force, offensive magic . . . while the expression *tama wahine,* "female side," covers everything that is contrary of these. . . . Man is sacred, woman is profane . . . "All evils, misery, and death," says a Maori proverb, "come from the female . . ."[8]

Again, need it be said which side is which?

Once out of the house and into the world of men, the left fares little better. Not even the pagan bacchanal is immune to the deadliest contamination from the forces of darkness locked in unholy alliance with the sinister. If by the merest chance you should find yourself knocking back a beer with a native on the Guinea coast, Hertz warns us, "watch his left hand, for the very contact of his left thumb with the drink would be sufficient to make it fatal."[9] Bottoms up, literally—with death waiting, as the Mexican Indian sorcerer Don Juan tells his Boswell, Carlos Casteneda, in that space to the immediate left of his frontward gaze.

In such societies as the Maori, furthermore, the equally high-priority masculine past times of warring and hunting are likewise taboo to the left:

What more sacred for primitive man than war or the hunt! . . . Is it possible to entrust something so precious to the left hand? This would be monstrous sacrilege, as much as it would be to allow a woman to enter the warriors' camp, i.e. to doom them to defeat and death. It is man's right side that is dedicated to the god of war; it is the *mana* of the right shoulder that guides the spear to its target; it is therefore only the right hand that will carry and wield the weapon.[10]

As if to give the back of his hand (the left, of course) to

our dim memory of the fearsome but luckless Benjamites, Hertz adds:

> The left hand, however is not unemployed: It provides for the needs of profane life that even an intense consecration cannot interrupt, and which the right hand, strictly dedicated to war, must ignore.[11]

What profane needs has Hertz in mind, we are left to wonder, that could stay the hand of Mars? Perhaps the Roman poet Martial and his absent ladies of the evening have the answer. Then again, maybe a latter-day communicator, artist-writer James De Kay (a left-hander) does. De Kay manfully faced what could be a close cousin of the same issue when he zeroed in on Arab eating habits in his bubbly little cartoon volume, *The Left-Handed Book.* The Arab custom of eating with the right hand—literally done with the fingers—he insists, has roots not in the theologic but in the hygienic.

"It stems solely from certain social problems that arise where water is scarce," says De Kay. We can almost see him swallow hard. "Some time back in history, they decided that the left hand should be reserved for certain . . . purposes, the intensely personal nature of which made that hand particularly unsuitable for the communal dinner pot."[12]

A more perfect metaphor for what society-at-large has always indicated man could do with his left hand can hardly be imagined.

Then again, hygiene can explain the primitive bias against the left hand no more than it can the civilized—witness this pagan ritual of the agrarian Mapuche Indians of Chile, which, shorn of its blood lust, sounds positively Christian in its dextral fixity:

The ritual priest . . . cuts off the right ear of the sacrificial sheep and holds it aloft in his right hand, while offering prayer to ancestors and the pantheon of Mapuche gods. The blood of the sheep is placed in a special wooden bowl to the right of the main altar. . . . Likewise, the sheep's heart is cut out and held aloft in the right hand of [the priest], who passes it to his chiefly assistants lined up along his right (and the right of the altar), who . . . bite into it, hold it up in their right hands, and offer ancestral prayer.[13]

Hindus use only the right hand to touch any part of their body above the navel, the left hand for any part below it. Bedouins segregate women to the left side of the tent, reserving the more illustrious right to the men. In rural Japan, left-handed women hide the fact lest they be found out and divorced. All in all, as Hertz and others of his ilk have found, there are scant exceptions to prove the auspicious rule of the dexter. Notable and almost alone are the Chinese, who consider the left a side of equal honor, and the American Zũni Indians, to whom the two sides personify brother gods of contrasting bent. To the Zũni, the left—surprise—is reflective, wise, and soundly judging. The right—surprise again—is impetuous, impulsive, and action-oriented.

Unspeakably primitive, you say? In a study of American school children from the first through ninth grades Domhoff found that negative feelings about the word "left" *increased steadily with age.* Three-year-olds in experimental play, moreover, used their dominant hand, usually the right, for socially acceptable activities and their nondominant hand, usually the left, for aggressive acts and—shades of the Hindu—intimate contact with their own bodies.

Most to the point, college freshmen and sophomores test-

46

ed by Domhoff on their subjective feelings about the words "left" and "right" overwhelmingly agreed with their more primitive brothers (and sisters) in the literature of anthropology. As Domhoff reports, the left was characterized by these sons and daughters of the technological twentieth century as bad, dark, profane, female, unclean, night, west, curved, limp, homosexual, weak, mysterious, low, ugly, black, incorrect, and death.

The right? Why, it was good, light, sacred, male, clean, day, east, straight, erect, heterosexual, strong, commonplace, high, beautiful, white, correct, and life.

In the face of such raging all-points mysticism, Hertz observed that philosophers have often recognized the distinction between left and right to be "one of the essential articles of our intellectual equipment."[14] As he perceptively concludes:

> It is clear that there is no question here of strength or weakness, of skill or clumsiness, but of different and incompatible functions linked to contrary natures. . . . The Power of the left hand is always somewhat occult and illegitimate; it inspires terror and repulsion. Its movements are suspect; we should like it to remain quiet and discreet, hidden in the folds of the garment, so that its corruptive influence will not spread. . . . Thus the belief in a profound disparity between the two hands sometimes goes as far as to produce a visible bodily asymmetry.[15]

Not only that, adds Hertz in his analysis of the prevailing human sentiment, "a left hand that is too gifted and agile is the sign of a nature contrary to right order, of a perverse and devilish disposition."[16] Its possessor, according to the universally dominant view, is "a possible sorcerer, justly to be distrusted."[17] ("Oh, I know the kind of people he's talking about," an artist friend of mine likes to interject at this point with mock brightness. "We call them nonconformists.")

To this stern indictment Hertz then adds a vital caveat:

This is why social selection favors right-handers and why education is directed to paralyzing the left hand while developing the right.[18]

Do we read him correctly? my artist friend and I demand almost in unison. Does Hertz mean to imply that society deliberately discriminates against the left hand in the absence of any real basis in neurophysiology, as Plato claimed—and does so to cement the polarity of its religious convictions?

Surveying the limited organic evidence available to him in the early 1900's, when even the incomplete neurology of my Dewey-dominated school days was still a generation away, Hertz answers with what amounts to a qualified yes: "Can one believe that a slight difference of degree in physical strength of the two hands could be enough to account for such a trenchant and profound [spiritual split in their symbolic significance]?"[19]

But why derogate the left and exult the right? Why not just as well do the opposite? Hertz asks himself the same pivotal question: ". . . the religious necessities which make the pre-eminence of one of the hands inevitable do not determine which of them will be preferred. How is it that the sacred side should invariably be the right and the profane the left?"[20]

Hertz duly rummages around in his intellectual equipment and dredges up a less-than-satisfactory reply. He puts it all down to that slight difference in manual strength—not congenital but conditioned, surely, he concedes—compounded across the ages by the social constraints of home care, etiquette, school and job training. Is that, we are impelled to ask, all? Not quite, Hertz amends. The whole is hitched to a qualitative judgment having its cause beyond the individual. But where? Why, in—*deus ex machina* to the rescue—the "collective consciousness" of man.[21]

Come now, Monsieur Hertz. That answer reminds me of the time an editor of a national magazine was asked by a California writer why it was published in New York and not, for example, in Los Angeles? After all his standard arguments had been defused and the editor realized he had been painted into a corner, he came up with an answer of stunningly existential import :

"Well . . . it has to be published *somewhere.*"

Granting the desperate thrust of Hertz's argument, symbolic manual primacy has to be invested *somewhere.* But the question goes begging. Why on the right? Why not, somewhere, sometime in civilized society, on the left?

Hertz covers his squidlike retreat from the field of speculation with a fusillade of bracketing remarks that, taken together, make a model of academic circularity:

The exclusive development of the right hand has sometimes been seen as a characteristic attribute of man and a sign of his moral preeminence. In a sense this is true. For centuries, the systematic paralyzation of the left arm has, like other mutilations, expressed the will animating man to make the sacred predominate over the profane, to sacrifice the desires and the interest of the individual to the demands felt by the collective consciousness and to spiritualize the body itself by marking upon it the opposition of values and the violent contrasts of the world on morality. . . .[22]

49

From there, of course, it is forensically easy sledding the rest of the way:

> A preponderant activity of the bad hand could only be illegitimate or exceptional; for it would be the end of man and everything else if the profane were ever allowed to prevail over the sacred and death over life. The supremacy of the right hand is at once an effect and a necessary condition of the order which governs and maintains the universe.[23]

"If organic asymmetry had not existed," declares Hertz, in man's time-honored salute to pragmatism, expediency, and convenience, "it would have had to be invented."[24]

But hold on. In the last analysis, could it be that we have done just that? Invented the sinister iniquities to appease some half-hidden imperative in our "collective consciousness"? And is it possible that this unspeakable *something* is more compatible at bottom with Jung's dark archetypes than with Hertz's placidly descriptive sociology, Judeo-Christian dogma, or the shining rationality that imbued the golden age of Greece?

Let us, before we bring the weight and light of modern science to bear, go back in time to a point before recorded history, in search of the illumination of further kinds of clues. Let us, in Domhoff's words, "stalk the artifacts of the unconscious."[25]

But first, a final ghostly word of Gallic caution from Robert Hertz to speed us on our way:

> The distinction of good and evil, which for long was [compatible] with the antithesis of right and left, will not vanish from our conscience the moment the left hand makes a more effective contribution to human labour and is able, on occa-

sion, to take the place of the right. If the constraint of a mystical ideal has for centuries been able to make man a unilateral being, physiologically mutilated, a liberated and foresighted community will strive to develop better the energies dormant in our left side . . . and to assure by an appropriate training a more harmonious development . . .[25]

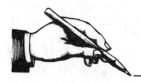

Tools of Conformity

4

More than two million years ago on the grassy savannas of deepest Africa, writes research psychologist Jerre Levy of the University of Pennsylvania, "an ape-like creature, low-browed and small-brained, stalked its prey—a young baboon. Having pigmy stature and flat humanoid teeth he might seem a poor challenge to [the baboon] with its vicious temper and lethal canines.

"But *Australopithecus* had a weapon—an antelope bone or fist-sized rock, and with it he crushed the baboon's skull."[1]

Typically, *Australopithecus,* regarded by most anthropologists as a forerunner of man, dragged his fallen prey back to his cave—where forensic pathologists less than three decades ago examined the skulls of the victims. Their skulls, Levy reports, revealed two significant findings. For one, the ancient baboon, like his successor,

failed to share with modern man one key anatomical characteristic—his skull was symmetrical, and did not show
certain enlarged areas on the left side. Equally important
for the purposes of our investigation, the baboon skulls
"showed not only that the crushing blow had been adminis-
tered quite deliberately with a weapon, but that the majority of the weapon wielders had been right-handed."[2]

These two asymmetries—modern man's skull configuration and his forerunner's hand use—"must reflect some important . . . step in the evolution of man,"[3] Levy concluded. But being a scientist, she carefully stopped short of
saying that one must cause the other, unlike H. G. Wells,
who once wrote, on the basis of lesser evidence, that man
was right-handed because the left side of his brain was bigger. And well Levy might hesitate. The evidence is tempting—irresistible to a man whose fictive imagination was to
inflame the minds of readers by the millions when it was
aimed finally at the unknowable future and not the exhuma-
ble past. But it is not conclusive. True, the left side of the
brain generally does govern the right side of the body, just
as the right side of the brain governs the body's left. And in
theory, there is every reason to suppose that if either side
of the brain were larger, it would have the greater oxygen
and blood supply and perhaps, thereby, a naturally denser
concentration of nerve fibers.

Indeed, we will discuss in detail later a similar theory of
nerve structure which is now one of the busiest avenues of
scientific inquiry into the nature of human handedness. All
of these factors conceivably could enable one side of our
brain, if larger, to cause a preference for the movement of
the hand it controls.

But outside *Australopithecus* the physical evidence remains mixed, meager, and indirect at best—so much so that

it would be rash to generalize as grandly as Wells. The reasons are several. For one, any historical perspective directly linking *Australopithecus* and modern man, leapfrogging as it does from one end of human time to the other, is limited. It overlooks, for example, the skulls of 700 Egyptians from the twenty-seventh to the thirtieth dynasty (525–332 B.C.) whose fossils were examined in 1929 and found to have a larger cerebral capacity in the *right* hemisphere. (As did the autopsied brain of the nineteenth-century German painter Adolph von Menzel, a left-hander.)

But most important, perhaps, such a hopscotch approach ignores the findings of archeology—the stuffed basement, attic, and hall closet of man's culture. With its tools, weapons, paintings, and writings it tells a different story. In their accumulation they indicate that handedness may have approached the fifty-fifty ratio of pure chance for Stone Age man, then dramatically shifted thereafter in favor of the dextral.

It may have done so, research suggests, for a complex of related reasons—reasons that have never, however, succeeded, with the weight of either logic or mysticism, in wiping the hated sinistral from the earth.

In the beginning, speaking archeologically and not Biblically, Paleolithic (Old Stone Age) man and his Neolithic (New Stone Age) successor survived by hunting, fishing, gathering edible plants, and, later, raising animals and farming by hoe. What crude tools and weapons they devised were fashioned from raw materials that existed in nature. Among them were bone, wood, antlers, ivory, or—most commonly, as the classification implies—stone.

Wells and Levy to the contrary, no strong collective preference for either hand is remotely evident in the rare remnants of Stone Age existence, which dates back over 5,000 years before Christ. Stone scrapers, hatchets, awls, borers, and flint pounders, unearthed from England to France and Switzerland, are almost evenly matched to either hand, most researchers have decided, when not actually interchangeable.

This does not mean, however, that prehistoric men had no individual preference—that they were, in fact, ambidextrous. "The evidence does not show that the same person had equal or divided dexterity," psychiatrist Abram Blau cautions in his book, *The Master Hand*. "It seems to point rather to a lack of a distinct differentiation of handedness."[4] Or as Sir Daniel Wilson, a left-handed Scottish archeologist who eventually taught himself to write with the right hand, declares in *The Prehistoric Man:*

> Every man did what was right in his own eyes. Some handled their tools and drew with the left hand. A larger number used the right hand, but as yet no rule prevailed. . . . Arts and habits . . . belonged to a chapter in the infancy of the race, when the law of dexterity . . . begot by habit, convenience or more prescriptive conventionality, had not yet found the place in that unwritten code to which a prompter obedience is rendered than to the most absolute of royal or imperial decrees.[5]

The law of dexterity, as Wilson terms it, was, in a manner of speaking, drafted, passed, and gradually instituted during the Bronze Age (3,000–1,000 B.C.). It was ratified with the invention of the wheel, the plow, the cart, writing, architecture, and—most important in Blau's view—bronze. Once man learned to produce and shape its hardness by smelting copper and alloying it with tin, a totally new and demanding world of multiple implements opened up. One might even say, Blau and other researchers would doubtless agree, that with it, true culture was born.

"The more complicated tools were better suited for one hand and had to be especially fashioned for such," contends Blau, like Wilson a left-hander. "Each tool certainly required great effort and much time to complete, and it was imperative for operators to use it with the hand for which it was constructed."[6] The shades of the Industrial Revolution rise up to haunt us as he adds, "The inventor or maker could decide the side of usage, whereas the user had little choice."[7]

Such a tool-based theory of handedness, Blau points out, is not only supported by the noticeably right-handed effects of wear and tear detected on the cutting edge of various Bronze Age implements. It is also backed by the discovery that the first sickles—as indeed the last—were almost exclusively designed for the dextral. According to archeologists, moreover, the oldest relics of early Sumerian and Egyptian culture, as well as their writing, arithmetic, and art, demonstrate the same right bias. (Early paintings show they wrote in exactly the way that would have done my old first grade teacher proud.)

Such a sturdy, well-wrought tool of tailored bronze, in Blau's words, "became a valuable possession, not too easily replaced, [one] handed down from generation to generation along with its dictates as to side of usage."[8]

With it, Blau goes on to claim, went inevitably a growing cultural need to prevent needless duplication, both of rare materials used and teaching effort expended. Such duplication, he thinks, could best be avoided by incorporating the skilled uniformity of hand into the social code. Thus codified, it could then be transmitted tribally with ever-growing authority down through the Iron Age to the present. All the moral, mythical, ethical, religious, and superstitious cant that has followed since with ever-increasing sophistication, Blau concludes, emerges "as a means of influencing people, of directing their behavior, of indoctrinating a preference."[9]

Parenthetically, Blau's emphasis on the cultural importance of tools as instruments of social conformity is indirectly buttressed by the relative nonconformism in more primitive societies, where tools are crude and scarce when not wholly nonexistent. A more or less equal distribution of handedness, if not outright sinister preference, still persists among savage cultures as diverse as the Bushmen, Hottentots, Australian aborigines, New Guineans, Bantus, and Pygmies. Judged by their arrowheads and spear blades, furthermore, the North American Indians once were a third sinistral.

Since the good/bad, right/left polarity holds for these pagans as well, it seems fair to conclude that the more sophisticated tools they come by, the more emphatic will become their insistence on a single hand, namely the right.

The act of writing evolved in much the same manner, Blau and other investigators would have it. While ancient language could be read from either direction, employing as it did pictographic signs instead of letters, when the Greeks borrowed the Phoenician alphabet, the rightful fate of Western writing was sealed forever. From the Semitic right-to-left orientation used by the Phoenicians, the Greeks switched first to—marvelous word—*boustrophedon*, a style in which lines were written and read down the page alternately in one direction, then the other, as a farmer plows the furrows of his field. (Boustrophedon means, literally, "as the ox turns.")

Finally the Greeks adopted left-to-right altogether. What proved culturally crucial about this, note French neurologists Henry Hécaen and Julian de Ajuriaguerra in their scientific book, *Left-Handedness: Manual Superiority and*

Cerebral Dominance, is that it was thereby "established in a people in which writing quickly became common to all social classes . . . [Writing] did not remain the exclusive privilege of priests or scribes."[10]

And with a preferred direction into the exclusive domain of the right hand, of course, went yet another task requiring the prolonged indoctrination of a highly specialized manual skill. Dextrality had become all the more democratic—made so by subtle mass pressures which, if more humane, were scarcely less effective in the long run than those of the Kaffirs and Indonesians. In childhood the Indonesian's left hand is completely bound to his side to discourage its use. When a Kaffir child's left hand grows too inquisitive, it is buried and scalded in the desert sand.

Persuasive as such anthropological findings are, however, they and the conclusions that Blau draw from them are by no means without dispute. Ancient art, for one thing, is not as clear-cut in its implications as Blau's argument might suggest. Agreed, Spanish cave drawings indicate a parity of Stone Age handedness, and later African cave art depicts a decided dextral bent. But we would be as wrong as Wells to leap to generalization. Sardinian invaders of pre-Christian Egypt are shown wearing shields on their right arms and wielding swords from their left. And for that matter, the Egyptians themselves—perhaps from the era of those larger right hemispheres in the brain?—are often pictured plowing, harvesting grain, and branding livestock in a manner that would make my wife decidedly uneasy because of the "awkwardness" she infers from my work in the kitchen.

Early literature is likewise conflicting. In addition to the scriptural account of the deadeye Benjamites, legend has it that Alexander the Great (356–323 B.C.) conquered a country whose inhabitants were left-handed and who accorded that hand the greater honor because it was anatomically nearer the heart.

As for the tools themselves, according to Hécaen and de Ajuriaguerra, among other critics, the only early implements which can be said with absolute conviction to be designed for one side and not the other are certain ones molded to fit the maker's hand, like the prehistoric scrapers of Alaska. Clearly, these are most often dextral.

Either way, the basic issue still goes begging: Why, in transmitting the cultural trappings of a saving conformity, did Bronze Age man, in most instances, always opt for the right hand, never the left? Can it really be a matter of pure chance? Given how widespread but isolated man's early remains are, it seems asking too much of chance that once random selection fell arbitrarily to the right in one place, it would then proceed to violate its very nature by endless repetition elsewhere. No, some natural principle must surely be operating. But what?

Blau believes that English essayist and historian Thomas Carlyle may have had the answer a century ago. Carlyle suspected the right may have gotten the upper hand, as it were, through something as simple as man's need to shield his heart in battle while wielding his weapon. Since his heart lay to the left, he protected it with that hand while fighting with his right—if he knew what was good for him. In the starkest kind of species selection, Carlyle suggests and Blau seconds, those who did may more often have come home carrying their shields, rather than being carried on them.

Even this, Hécaen and de Ajuriaguerria sharply question. Women, they reasonably point out, did not bear arms, yet they have become even more right-handed than men.

Then too, the shield or buckler did not originate as a passive method of protecting the heart, but rather derives from a stick or baton used aggressively to parry an opponent's blows. To manipulate it effectively, they argue, required a manual strength and skill at least equal to that of the weapon hand.

No one, however—not mystic, priest, anthropologist, archeologist, psychologist, sociologist, neurophysiologist, teacher, or interested left-hander—can quarrel with Blau's linchpin observation:

"The obvious fact [is] that despite all the training to which they are exposed, left-handed children still appear. Notwithstanding the pressures brought to bear on them, many persist. . . ."[11]

So in the end, it appears, why man prefers the right remains as much a mystery as why the left persists in the face of practically everything. Both questions however, share a common ground, and perhaps there is where we should look for our answers. Whatever the reason, in everything he does, *man does demonstrate a preference.* Is he alone in his sidedness? we must ask ourselves. And if he is not, what else in the physical world shares his curious idiosyncrasy (if that is what it is), and what can we learn from it?

Nature awaits. Let us go and see.

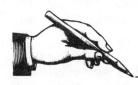

Through a Glass Looking

5

To most of us, the natural world appears made of elemental matter that has no fundamental preference for one hand or the other. Stars spin either way. So do the whorls of seashells. Only man as a species, we believed—erroneously, in a sense, as we shall see—only man among all things living prefers the right to the left.

A few of us, of course, may have heard vaguely of left- and right-handed molecules, but the terms seemed at best a scientific technicality. The idea of a cosmic preference, much less what this might mean to humans of either manual persuasion, was scarcely something you talked about at cocktail parties. Indeed, as recently as 1957 the nature of life on earth demonstrated no underlying material bias to either the left or right that we understood as such. Whatever spun, whorled, turned, moved, grew, or displayed in any other physical manner a distinct preference for one hand could—or so scientists thought—just as easily do so for the opposite. If it did not, we had only to look more closely at ramified nature to find its antithesis, its mirror image.

At least, that appeared unshakably true in principle. The universe, or so we imagined, was ambidextrous—in theory, if not always in fact. That concept, called parity, was one of the mainstays of physics, a crucial crossbeam in the scaffolding upon which our oh-so-patiently put-together structure of supposedly immutable natural laws was erected.

Then, in a cold shower of electrons, everything changed. And we saw, or at least physicists did to their everlasting consternation, that our very planet itself, the cradle of all terrestrial existence, could have a basic preference for one hand. No magician had ever demonstrated such consummate legerdemain.

How? While a case of microscopic hairsplitting, the answer is worth our examination because it suggests—as does one eminent neurophysiologist—that human handedness could actually be shaped by natural forces in the outside world. Farfetched as such an idea may appear at first glance, if he is correct, these forces are no less powerful for being all but invisible to our naked eye.

That nature in its manifold workings exhibits many forms of handedness, if not a readily apparent preference for one hand over the other, is hardly worth debating, though some are far less obvious than others. We know, for instance, as Martin Gardner points out in his marvelous book *The Ambidextrous Universe,* that the magnetic axis of the sun now and again, for reasons we don't understand, does a flip-flop. Plus becomes minus, each pole the other. In effect, although its spin stays the same, the sun changes hands.

Closer to home, as Gardner goes on to relate, we are indebted to a nineteenth-century French engineer named Gaspard Gustave de Coriolis for discovering the pronounced form of planetary handedness that bears his name. Because the earth spins, he found, it imparts to its surface movement a torque strong enough to determine the prevailing twist of tornadoes, cyclones, ocean currents and—just maybe—water draining out of your bathtub. In other words, since the southern hemisphere of the globe spatially mirrors the northern hemisphere (with the equator as its dividing line), the Coriolis effect tends to cause the whirlpool-like vortices of all such phenomena to twist clockwise north of the equator, counterclockwise south of it. In a rough sense, therefore, each hemisphere is to the other as the left hand is to the right.

Though not always even that evident, the immediate macroscopic natural world of physical matter around us shares an outward if static evenhandedness that scientists call *theoretical symmetry.* This symmetry, or lack of hand preference, must remain theoretical because, while often visible and obvious, it is sometimes neither. To understand how handedness applies to this aspect of nature, we must understand both kinds, the existing and hypothetical, the kind we can see and the kind we cannot. For unless we do, human handedness will remain nothing more than an incidental curiosity.

To take the visible and obvious first, such symmetry (evenhandedness) is apparent in objects that are bilateral in shape about a vertical axis. That is, they have two identical but complementary sides (or hands). *Bilateral symmetry,* as it is called, abounds in nature for a powerful reason, so obvious it almost evades our awareness altogether: gravity. Gravity makes lakes spread and hold to the earth, mountains pyramid ever smaller from their massive foundations, trees reach out from their clinging roots to put forth limbs in a contour rudely conical.

Disparate matter and form though they be, bodies of water, growing wood, and the upthrusting earth are all ruled by the same spatial dynamic—one that makes it possible for us, in theory anyway, to draw an infinite number of symmetrical planes through their surface vertically, none at all horizontally. (Figure 1). We can take endless cross-sections that are roughly identical if we cut them through the vertical axis like a birthday cake, not even as many as two if we attempt to slice them sidewise. The reason is simple. They have no horizontal axis. (A birthday cake, being cylindrical or rectangular, has both kinds, vertical and horizontal, but only one of the latter.)

Thus these natural objects—lakes, trees, and mountains—are said to be evenhanded, to have bilateral symmetry about a vertical axis. Or put another way, their sides match, but their tops and bottoms don't. Most visible and obvious symmetry in nature falls into this category.

There is, however, a larger kind of symmetry in nature which includes the visible and obvious but is not limited to it. In fact, in its strictest sense such evenhandedness is not only invisible to the unaided eye, it frequently exists only in the hypothetical sense of the word, which is why we call it theoretical symmetry.

As Martin Gardner explains it, this less-than-obvious natural symmetry can easily be verified by holding a sample scene of outdoors terrain up to a mirror. Here, the *mirror image* provides the opposing "hand" needed to create a symmetry that is bilateral. The vertical axis, of course, is the interface of mirror and reality. Shown the reflection alone, we see nothing that could not just as readily exist. Ergo, physicists would argue, it has theoretical symmetry.

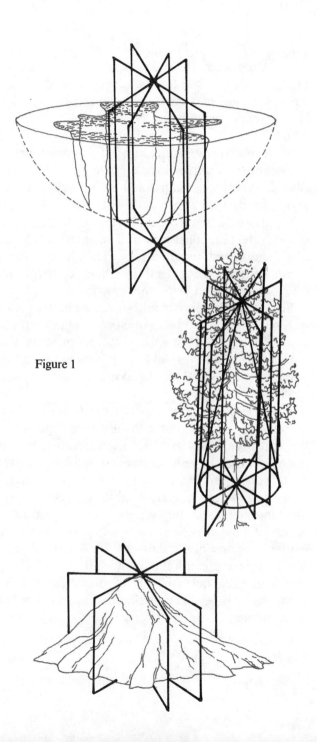

Figure 1

Viewed together, the sides, tops, and bottoms all match. The positions of the trees are reversed, yes, the clouds in the sky switched spatially, the reeds in the lake made to bloom magically out of the left shallows instead of the right. But nothing in the reflection is impossible or nonsensical. If the lake were clear and still enough, in fact, the entire scene-plus-mirror-image could be visually turned upside down, the actuality and its reflection reversed, and none would be the wiser.

Naturally, if this were a movie, and a rock were dropped in the water, the illusion would be shattered. Such a trick is often employed by directors. They shoot the reflection rather than the scene itself and then destroy it, both to capture our attention with the unexpected and to comment obliquely on the perishability of life and the transitoriness of time. What could be more surprising, or more profoundly disturbing, than the apparent disintegration of ostensible reality before our very eyes? The power of such an effect is a measure of how persuasive the mirror-image illusion can be.

A movie projectionist with a subtle sense of the absurd, moreover, can drive home the illusionary persuasiveness of the mirror image even more emphatically simply by threading his film so the light shines through from the wrong side. As Gardner points out, "You might watch such a film for some time before you realized it had been flopped."[1] Run the film backward, though, as he says, and the unearthly antics of time reeling in reverse are hilariously and amply evident, as any home moviemaker knows. Cars run backward, divers are miraculously spit out of the swimming pool and back onto the diving board, assembly lines become marvels of dismantlement. Time cannot fool us; not here, anyway.

But we are fooled by mirror images because, as long as theoretical symmetry holds, what the mirror can create, nature can duplicate. Unless the scene is familiar to us, this supremely plausible reversal—what amounts to nothing less than a change of hand—fails to look strange.

Introduce man-made objects into the picture, however, and this mirror symmetry can be spoiled in a way nature normally does not duplicate. Not that this always happens. By and large, man aesthetically prefers patterns that have the same sort of evenhandedness that infuses nature. Perhaps, Gardner suggests, this is why it pleases us so. Possibly because gravity is such a pervasive sculpting factor in our lives, we work bilateral symmetry into almost everything we make: cubistic buildings, rectilinear streets and sidewalks, cruciform telephone poles. When mirror-imaged, the two sides reflect symmetrically, just as they do in nature. If anything, they are infinitely more precise in their match. They merely change places and, being complementary, assume each other's identity, like perfect twins or a pair of hands. Everything is switched, nothing extrinsic is changed.

However, most man-made objects lacking bilateral symmetry can be tripped up by the mirror, right? Wrong. Like the rest of visible nature, they retain at least a theoretical symmetry when reflected, because their mirror-image loses no meaning and consequently contributes the missing "hand" that completes the bilaterality. Inserting either a rectangular mailbox or a motorcycle into our mirrored landscape, for instance, fails to spoil the scene's theoretical symmetry. The mailbox, being relatively two-sided and reversible on its vertical axis, already *has* an evenhandedness. Its bilateral symmetry is unaffected, really, by mirroring. The motorcycle does not have an evenhandedness, and

69

is affected by mirroring. Its front and back clearly differ, but its mirror-image makes as much visual sense as the object itself. Therefore it completes the bilaterality, and theoretical symmetry is preserved.

But can't everything, then, have a mirror image? Haven't we just proved that theoretical symmetry is inviolable, in man as well as nature?

We haven't, not by a long shot. We need do only one small thing to our assembled landscape to destroy its theoretical symmetry, its hypothetical evenhandedness, forever: *print a name on either object, mailbox or motorcycle.* The letters are reversed, all right, a mirror image is maintained, but the result *no longer makes sense.* For language is the one asymmetric element in human culture obvious, persuasive, and compelling enough to cancel out consistently our built-in propensity for the bilateral.

Indeed, any such sign, relying as it does on the linear, one-directional thrust of language for its meaning, will tell us very quickly when the evenhandedness of theoretical symmetry has been violated. In photography, for example, we know instantly that we are looking at a color transparency from the wrong, or mirror, side if the lettering on the subject's tee shirt, say, looks more like the Cyrillic alphabet of the Russians than our own and is about as readable.

Naturally, someone could produce such mirror-lettered tee shirts as a novelty. Probably someone has. Mirror-writing and -reading is a fascinating game for children; usually it is the first "code" they learn. But the point still stands: There is nothing natural about it. If we see such a language reversal, we grasp its implication at once. If the shirt in the picture is unlettered, we may never know.

On a sportcoat, though, the sharp of mind and eye would

spot the switch instantly, whether or not the wearer's name was embroidered over the breast pocket. Why? Because the coat would appear to be buttoned on the wrong, that is to say, the female, side. For the social dictates of custom in clothing are as asymmetric as language.

(One theory has it that this sartorial difference in the sexes originated from the same cause: our prevailing history of right-handedness. Women of style-setting nobility were dressed by their maids, who, being predominantly right-handed, found it easier to button the garment from right to left. Men, in contrast, dressed themselves—and came to prefer the opposite arrangement of buttons all the more because it enabled them to keep their weapon hand warmed for action by stuffing it into their blouse. Unfortunately, neither fact gets us any nearer to solving the riddle of why people, in the old days, were right-handed.)

What all this means, of course, is that where it exists, man's lack of symmetry is either obvious or can be made apparent. The preferred hand of his works can be exposed by the simple use of a mirror. Nature, as it happens, is something else again. While nature's theoretical symmetry might seem invincibly absolute, at its deepest depths that symmetry is anything but absolute, a fact which resists revelation in all but the most exquisite subatomic experimentation.

Indeed, to go back a bit, the handedness it expresses at the higher molecular level of matter—sometimes left, sometimes right, sometimes both—is random, inconclusive in its thrust, and usually present in complementary forms. It is likewise subtle. But both kinds of asymmetry, that found in molecules and that found in subatomic particles, nevertheless conceivably contribute in some as-yet-unex-

71

plained fashion to a physical world which may draw forth an answering asymmetry in the handedness of man.

To see how this might be possible, let us go on to explore these unseen realms, whose essential handedness was for so long unknown and unsuspected.

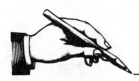

Twisting the Light Fantastic

6

Consider the curious case of crystals, the solid stuff of nonlife—and some life—itself. Crystals are at the top of the atomic ladder that governs all structure. They are the repeating three-dimensional patterns into which the molecules of most purely solid inanimate matter are arranged. These patterns apply equally to the geometric building blocks of such diverse solids as snow, salt and diamonds. A crystal's *lattice* is the Tinker Toy-like configuration of atoms or molecules that give it such distinctive patterns (Figure 2).

Generally cubical in form, the crystal lattice can have any number of sides or faces. It can be symmetrical (even-handed) or—in that most common of minerals, quartz—asymmetrical (Figure 3). Quartz, for that matter, can be thought of as either left-handed or right-handed, as many crystals can, because the structure of their lattice twists

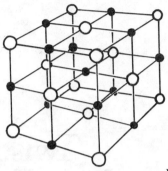

Figure 2

more or less into a fantastically elaborate corkscrew whose threads can go either way (Figure 4).

Early in the last century it was discovered that quartz does a funny thing to light—an inadvertent key that further unlocked the mysterious handedness of the universe. Because its intricate crystalline structure acts as a baffle, clear quartz, when bombarded by a beam of light, allows it to penetrate only along a single plane. Then, depending on how its corkscrew pattern is threaded, it twists the light in that direction, either right or left, giving us a relatively simple visual method of determining whether its lattice is right- or left-handed.

Moving a microscopic step further, scientists next asked if the molecules of matter *themselves* might have a basic, if unseen, handedness. Like quartz crystals, could they be aligned into either one of a double set of mirror images physically identical in all respects except handedness? And if so, what would this mean, assuming it meant anything at all, to the basic constituency and function of the matter it comprised?

The first question and its ultimate answer fell to Louis Pasteur, the father of pasteurization. Then a young and unknown chemist just starting his career, Pasteur knew that quartz crystals failed to twist light when they were dissolved in solution. That must mean the lattice, their geometric structure, was critical; the light-twisting property of quartz resided there and not within the molecules themselves.

Pasteur knew, too, on the other hand, that certain organic compounds were also "optically active," as the phenomenon is described, *in solution and without benefit of a crystalline lattice.* In their case the twist had to be embedded in the structure of the molecule; there was no place else it could be. Finally, Pasteur knew another significant thing about one such compound found in grapes—tartaric acid. It existed in another form called racemic acid, which was identical down to but excluding one last vital detail: It did not twist light.

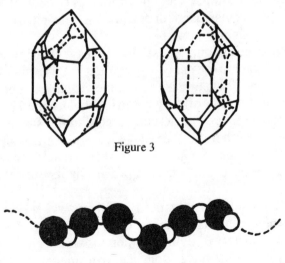

Figure 3

Figure 4

"Here was a curious situation indeed," writes Martin Gardner. "How can two things be exactly alike in all respects, yet differ in the way they transmit light? Pasteur could imagine only one explanation. . . . There must be some sort of left-right difference in the structure of the molecules."[1]

Putting tartaric acid crystals under his microscope, Pasteur quickly saw what we, if not he, might have expected: They were uniformly asymmetrical in the same direction. In short, they had a single handedness. In contrast, the crystals of racemic acid, when magnified, stood revealed as *a precisely equal mixture of left- and right-handed molecules* which, in their optical effect, baffled one another, cancelled each other out, so to speak.

Scrupulously separated with miniature tools, however, the two kinds of molecules not only passed every chemical test for tartaric acid, each twisted light *the opposite way.* They were, in sum, exact mirror images of each other.

Was molecular handedness just a nuclear parlor trick or did it truly signify something?

Pasteur could only guess. But he saw clearly the importance of the mirror image to symmetry: "The simultaneous production of two opposite asymmetric halves is equivalent to the production of a symmetric whole, whether the two asymmetric halves be actually united in the same molecule . . . or whether they exist as separate molecules, as in the left and right constituents of racemic acid. In any case, the symmetry of the whole is proved by its optical inactivity."[2]

Now, thanks to advances in chemistry, we know that such molecular handedness does have functional meaning—in a variety of living compounds which either exist dually in nature or have atomic mirror images which can be synthesized in the laboratory—often to opposite, if not always rewarding, ends. For although their right- and left-handed forms respond indifferently to the buffetings of such unbiased elemental forces as temperature and gravity (and why not, since they are—almost—identical?), they frequently reveal their essential difference in important ways.

According to Gardner, for example, the dextral mirror image of sinister Vitamin C is almost an outright placebo. It scarcely affects us at all. Nor does the milder right-handed brother molecule of (levo) nicotine. Unfortunately for smokers, (dextro) nicotine can only be concocted in the lab; the tobacco of nature is stuck with the more harmful form. (A dextro-cigarette would not only cost much more across the counter initially, given the economics of marketing, it's an odds-on bet to smell and taste different too, and probably not for the better.)

Similarly, Gardner tells us, if you reverse the left-handed versions of natural adrenaline and hyoscyamine—a glandular blood vessel constrictor and eye-dilating alkaloid, respectively—you rob them of their powers. Conversely, switch hands synthetically on the sinister hormone thyroxine, and its ability to cut cholesterol is retained while the side effects of weight loss and nervousness are reduced. Finally—and we needn't don a lab coat to capitalize on it—dextrose, or (right-handed) grape sugar, is sweeter yet less harmful to diabetics than levulose, or (left-handed) fruit sugar.

All of these effects, apparently, and perhaps many more yet to be found, depend on nothing more complicated (or less complex) than which way their molecules twist.

Most intriguing of all, in strictly human terms, is the handedness of protein—the highest chemical expression of that common denominator to all life, carbon in compound. Carbon is the most pervasive substance on earth. With its potentially endless, infinitely ramified chaims—a "charm bracelet," in Gardner's words, of godlike proportions—carbon can take literally *billions* of animate forms. Protein in the human body alone assumes an estimated one hundred thousand different varieties. Within these highly complex forms, any two molecules may be exactly alike in number, kind, and arrangement of atoms, yet be *structural mirror images of each other.* These are called *stereoisomers* (from the Greek for three-dimensionally "of like parts"). They can exist by the tens of thousands in giant carbon molecules having an asymmetric pattern.

As it happens, the most numerous of these are proteins, but here a word of semantic caution: A stereoisomer's mirror image need not actually exist, within the molecule or outside of it. If only by definition, it exists in theoretical symmetry, a ghostly reflected doppelgänger embodied by concept, just as our reflection can be said to "exist" without the constant presence of a mirror to see it.

The distinction is important because—as majority members of our essentially right-handed society may be mildly distressed to learn—*virtually every protein in all living things, humans included, is a left-handed stereoisomer.*

Putting aside for the moment just why this should be so, we know that our body, whether we be popping medicinal pills or wining and dining, is innately gifted with a wondrous if mystifying capacity to discriminate chemically between left- and right-handed stereoisomers. It may digest both at different rates, or digest one and excrete the other. We are not unique in this. So it is with all plants and animals.

A decade after his first great discovery, Pasteur contributed a second penetrating insight into the elemental handedness of matter along exactly those lines. He reported that racemic acid could be rendered optically active without the busy intercession of a sorting human hand. How? By growing in it a certain plant mold, one which was found to devour selectively all the molecules of one handedness, thus liberating those of the other to exercise their native light-twisting ability.

Being an asymmetric living organism, he wrote, the mold

> selects for its nutriment that particular form of tartaric acid which suits its needs—the form, doubtless, which in some way fits its own asymmetry . . . [It] exhibits a power which no symmetrical chemical substance, such as our ordinary oxidizing agents, and no symmetric form of energy, such as heat, can ever possess: It distinguishes between [stereoisomers.][3]

Pasteur's subsequent studies led him to conclude, moreover, that while most molecules in any form of life are asymmetric and have one handedness or the other, but not both, nonliving molecules, when asymmetric, invariably have racemic or mixed handedness. Hence, though the living are usually active optically and twist light (because they are on balance asymmetric), the nonliving molecules never do. The equal presence of both kinds of handedness within the same inanimate molecule, he decided, creates an overall symmetry that destroys either directional torque.

That this telling boundary exists between the animate and inanimate may be obvious, but what it tells us is not. Pasteur suspected the distinction was critical and lay at the hidden heart of life itself: "I am on the verge of mysteries, and the veil which covers them is getting thinner and thinner,"[4] he wrote a friend. He felt life was "a function of the asymmetry of the universe and of the consequences of this fact"[5]—consequences most certainly derived from asymmetric forces in the prehistoric environment which stirred the primordial soup of earthly existence into a rich and bubbly broth somehow inseparable from the thrust that gave it vital direction.

But even as we nod to Pasteur and acknowledge that direction to be surprisingly sinistral, how are we to account for its generative thrust? Left-handed at bottom life may be, but why, and to what end?

Twentieth-century science, while confirming most of Pasteur's empirical conclusions, is helpless to answer. "To this day," Gardner concedes, "no one knows how the first . . . half-living molecules got their particular handedness."[6] Inanimate asymmetric compounds, scientists have decided, are racemic because left- and right-handed molecules are evenly distributed by the blind, impartial workings of sheer chance, the random force that operates in keeping with the law of equal probability, for example, every time you flip a coin. Eventually, we know, heads will turn up as often as tails, but only eventually, in some larger sample. To achieve such a natural balance, inanimate matter has had literally all the time in the world. But what about living molecules? In the beginning of life, why was chance summarily repealed, probability tilted until it became the inevitable?

Biochemists offer several hypothetical explanations, all of them variations on the same cosmic theme: *Something happened* (perhaps at the outset only a paper-thin 51–49 shave in probability odds) to give the sinister molecule of life-giving carbon the upper hand. Self-replicated across the geologic ages, they think, that slight numerical advantage exponentially converted itself at last to ironclad genetic mastery.

Again, is this important? For determining human handedness, in and of itself, it is probably not. Most neuroscientists would doubtless agree with one leading researcher who dismisses molecular sinistrality as totally irrelevant to macroscopic events. Man and other cellular constellations of sinister stereoisomers, as we have seen, can replicate themselves out of nutrients having either handedness—and from even-handed compounds as well. After all, plants manufacture asymmetric starches from symmetric molecules of water and carbon dioxide. From the atom up, we look in vain at human protein for any extrinsic sign of a structural imperative having impact upon which hand we are to use in wielding a fork or pencil.

Besides, if there *were* a significant but as yet undetected correlation, why would it express itself in a predominantly right-handed way, yet still leave room for a sizable minority of left-handers? If some people were at base made of left-handed molecules and others of right—in any sort of apt ratio, crossed or not—the proposition might make more empirical sense. As it is, it remains the remotest sort of speculation.

Within the dervishly whirling heart of the atom, however, lurks still another unexpected asymmetry, one so elemental that, taken together with the molecular, it conceivably could reflect something in the laws of motion decisive in determining which hand we prefer to use.

Down with Parity (Whatever It Is)

7

The fall of parity—the shattering of our nuclear mirror—is so rich in requisite detail, so far-ranging in possible ramification, that it all but defies understandable brevity. For those who wish to know more about the many episodes that make up this rousing if Lilliputian adventure in particle physics, Martin Gardner's exhaustive and lucid account in *The Ambidextrous Universe* is recommended without reservation. For now, we will confine ourselves to the profound meaning of one unprecedented experiment, the results of which have smashed forever the faith in science in an even-handed world.

As traditionally viewed by the physicist, life as we know it is based on three interlocking principles of symmetry, critical dimensions of existence which apart or in combination seem inviolable when attempting to explain the universe.

83

These are fixed points of reference, absolutes, the presumed *sine qua non* of our existence.

One, of course, is the evident symmetry of reflection, the seemingly axiomatic assumption that any event as it is seen in a mirror could just as easily occur that way as it did in actuality. A second, less apparent, symmetry is that of electric charge, which, as imbued in atomic structure, can be either plus or minus. The third symmetry—and the least apparent—is, curiously enough, the all-saturating one of time.

All of these—in theory at any rate—were thought to be reversible. If the one reflection was obvious, the other two were decidedly less so. Clearly, reality and its mirror image could be reversed with nothing materially altered but handedness. Indeed, at the molecular level, we have learned that left- and right-handed stereoisomers are quite common. Less obvious is the fact that any plus charge in the constituency of matter can be minus, and vice versa. Mutual annihilation would ensue instantly from our contact with such "antimatter," to be sure, since all matter would instantly be converted to energy in a massive chain reaction, but science fiction has taught us there is no physical reason why antimatter should not exist safely somewhere off in the cosmos across a buffer of limitless space.

Finally, fantastic as it might seem (outside science fiction anyway), physicists unflappably agreed that "time's arrow" itself could be reversed. That is, time could literally run backward instead of forward. And why not? "It is not time that flows but the world," writes Gardner.[1]

Strictly speaking, there is nothing in the laws of nature to prevent that movement from happening in reverse. "There is only," Gardner adds, "the difficulty of imagining how it could get started."[2]

Nevertheless, in "Can Time Go Backward?"—an article

he wrote years ago for *Scientific American*—Gardner had great fun in trying his hand at just such an exercise in "time invariance," as it is known, one employing the mundane mechanics of the pool table:

A cue ball breaks a triangle of 15 balls on a pool table. The balls scatter hither and thither and the 8 ball, say, drops into a side pocket. Suppose immediately after this event the motions of all the entities involved are reversed in direction while keeping the same velocities. At the spot where the 8 ball came to rest the molecules that carried off the heat and shock of impact would all converge on the same spot to create a small explosion that would start the ball back up the incline. Along the way the molecules that carried off the heat of friction would move toward the ball and boost it along its upward path. The other balls would be set in motion in a similar fashion. The 8 ball would be propelled out of the side pocket and the balls would move around the table until they finally converged to form a triangle. There would be no sound of impact because all the molecules that had been involved in the shock waves produced by the initial break of the triangle would be converging on the balls in such a way that the impact would freeze the triangle and shoot the cue ball back toward the tip of the cue.[3]

Although such a macroscopic event would look every bit as funny on film as the time reversals mentioned in an earlier chapter, "a motion picture of any individual molecule . . . would show absolutely nothing unusual. No basic mechanical law would seem to be violated."[4]

Given the billions of molecules precisely involved in such a transaction, however, Gardner hastens to emphasize that the chance of such a happening is so slight as to be all but inconceivable.

At that, it is a mere microcosm of what would need to occur at the point of impact to reassemble and propel back into orbit any of the thousands of meteorites that have struck the earth since time—or should we say the planet?—began. Still, in both cases, the macroscopic and the telescopic, the barrier is statistical, not physical; one of probability, not possibility.

As far as the direction of time's winged arrow was concerned, provided the initial conditions existed at its perimeter to turn such a radiative process around—a Herculean proviso—the reverse sequence could not help but occur. Together with the symmetries of reflection and charge, time symmetry was, or so physicists thought, one of nature's inalienable laws.

Where—and what—was parity in all this?

Parity refers to the reflection principle, the conservation law that says nature is blind to any difference between left and right in its fundamental workings. Conservation, in turn, simply implies that its blindness endures, its lack of an overriding preference never changes. As Gardner cautions, "This does not mean that asymmetry cannot turn up in the universe in all sorts of ways.

"It only means that anything nature does in a left-handed way, she can do just as easily and efficiently in a right-handed way"[5]—just as time in some other galaxy conceivably could move backward instead of forward.

So we have seen with molecules. The quantities in each pair of stereoisomers need not be equal. Both need not even palpably *be*. Their qualitative existence (as with antimatter, in the comfortably distant realm of theory alone) is sufficient.

Practically speaking, the proof of parity in all its ostensibly unswerving reliability of reflection can be demonstrated in something as simple as the phenomenon of odd and even numbers. As any school child quickly learns, an even number added to another even number always produces a number that is even, as does an odd number added to another odd number. This, to complicate things, is called *even parity.*

Conversely, when an even and an odd number are added, the result is always an odd number. This is called *odd parity.* No matter how large or small the numbers involved, either pattern will invariably yield the predicted result, like a mirror reflecting.

In other words, parity, odd or even, is always conserved. To flog the point to the edge of extinction, add odd *or* even numbers and you get a number that is even: *even parity.* Add odd *and* even numbers, on the other hand, and you get a number that is odd: *odd parity.* Never in the recorded history of man had anybody, in effect, added two even numbers and gotten *an even number one time, an odd number the next.*

Never, that is, until the astonishing advent of what physicists term the "theta tau puzzle."

In 1956 scientists discovered to their bewilderment that a strange subatomic particle called the K-meson was showing them the nuclear equivalent of the two faces of Janus, that ancient Roman god of the gates whose twin faces looked in opposite directions.

One of these "faces," called the theta meson, decayed during its oh-so-brief burst of life (one ten-billionth of a second, laggard for a particle) into two particles called pi mesons. What was believed to be the other face, or form, of the K-meson, the tau meson, decayed into *three* pi mesons.

87

In all other vital respects theta and tau were identical. Yet the difference was critical, and befuddling, because both the theta meson and the pi meson were known to have, in a technical sense far too abstruse to be dealt with here, *even parity.*

Since tau decomposed into three pi mesons instead of two, it could hardly have the same parity as theta. Although theta and tau were clearly not mirror images of each other, could they be two different particles, one with even parity, the other with uneven? Implausible as that seemed at such an infinitesimal level of matter, the alternative was unthinkable: that theta and tau were one and the same, a K-meson which sometimes decayed into two pi mesons and other times into three, in blithe and flouting disregard for the sanctity of universal even-handedness.

If that were so, parity was not conserved. Far from it. It was a cosmic crap game.

In 1957 came just such a momentous disclosure. First, two young Chinese physicists working in the United States, Chen Ning Yang and Tsing-Dao Lee, were awarded the Nobel prize for their discovery that *no evidence existed* for conservation of parity in weak interactions—of which the theta tau puzzle seemed only the most flagrant violation. Then along came the world's most eminent woman physicist, their colleague Madame Chien-Shiung Wu of Columbia University, to prove the unthinkable experimentally.

Cooling a radioactive isotope of cobalt down to near absolute zero (-273 degrees centigrade) and thereby stilling the isotope's jittery molecules, she next applied an electromagnetic field inducing their electrons to be shot out either north or south. Then she sat back to watch how many of them went each way.

If the number divided equally in this characteristically weak interaction and decay, all would be well. Indirectly it would mean that parity had held, that theta and tau were not the same K-meson, that the apprehendable universe remained in theory ambidextrous.

But no, most of the electrons promptly went south, bearing with them the cherished and long-standing conviction of nuclear science that we live in an elementally symmetrical and balanced physical world. Parity did not hold. In weak interactions, nature as we knew it harbored a secret hand preference. For which? Need you ask? It was just as one of the giants of physics, Wolfgang Pauli, had feared: "The Lord was a weak left-hander."[6]

Thirty years before, Hungarian physicist Eugene Wigner had demonstrated to the satisfaction of physics that all forces involved in particle interaction were evenhanded, that is, reflectable in parity's mirror. Now Madame Wu in one fell stroke had proved this simply wasn't so. In mundane terms, a motion picture of her classic experiment, when run in reverse through a projector, would be, in Gardner's words, "a picture of an experiment which could not be performed anywhere in the galaxy."[7]

The scientific community was as stunned as a lay audience would be if in Gardner's hypothetically reversed pool shot the film had shown the scattered balls reassembling themselves on the table in a *vertical* triangle, one on top of the other, like the human pyramid formed by acrobats in a circus.

Since then, the other principles of symmetry in some of their separate or combined dimensions have buckled under renewed experimental assault. But while enormously significant, and troubling, to our ultimate understanding of nature's laws, their exposed or suspected flaws need not directly concern us here, where handedness is the issue. Only one more pivotal question, in fact, need be asked before moving briskly on to examine handedness in higher forms of life:

Granted its fundamental importance to the minute world of particle physics, how could anything so miniscule as the violation of parity in weak subatomic interactions—profoundly basic to the structure of all matter as it admittedly is—act to influence, much less determine, which hand we as humans tend to prefer?

Perhaps Wigner has the seeds of an answer:

> One can conclude that the laws of nature do show a preference for either the right or the left hand. We are surrounded by many phenomena that appear to show such a preference, or more precisely, such a distinction between right and left. Most of us are right-handed and our hearts are on the left side. On a large scale we observe that the earth rotates to the left (counterclockwise) as seen from above the North Pole and proceeds to the left around the sun. The sun, in turn, travels to the right around the galaxy as viewed from above the north galactic pole.
>
> Heretofore these asymmetries were attributed to asymmetries in the initial conditions. *Now it is possible to attribute the same asymmetries to the laws of motion, that is, to assume that the universe was initially more symmetrical than it is now and that the present state evolved as a result of the asymmetry of the laws of motion.*[8]

In 1956, when he first offered these rather freewheeling speculations, Wigner was quick to concede that few people were ready to entertain them seriously, himself included. But if such elemental asymmetry exists in the laws of motion, it seems sensible to ask, why should their effects be confined to the microscopic?

Let us pursue this tantalizing question on up into the kingdom of flora and fauna, to see if any further clues to such a cosmic handedness can be found there.

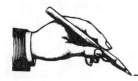

Bindweed
and Anableps

8

Do plants and animals demonstrate anything like the hand preference of human beings? Do they behave as if the elemental laws of motion in any way invest them with an overpowering asymmetry of shape and movement?

The answer is yes, no, and maybe. Taking the smallest and simplest things first, both forms of life, plant and animal, in the beginning evolved from one-celled organisms tossing on the ocean's surface in buoyant, spherical disregard for even the most rudimentary spatial orientation. They were like the perfect, symmetrical men of Greek myth. They cared nothing for up and down, much less for front and back or—a quantum leap up the scale of directional coordinates—left and right.

But, notes Gardner, as soon as early plants began to attach themselves to the ocean floor, a permanent up-down axis was created that in due time carried over to rooting on land. Growing in the relatively open-ended space of sea or air, neither of which required of them any obvious lateral differentiation, plants generally came to develop the crude symmetry of the cone or cylinder when not (fruits especially) the sphere.

There are, of course, important exceptions, examples of structural asymmetry with intriguing implications almost metaphoric in their significance. These are the climbing, twining plants which coil in graceful helices, the right- or left-handed woodscrew configuration common, if complexly so, to crystal lattices and molecules. Remember the helix. We will meet it again when we come to the human brain.

Some helical species, like the honeysuckle, twist left. Others, like the morning glory and other bindweeds, twist right. Still others twist either way. The chaotic mess when helical plants of opposite bent embrace each other through an accident of nature is almost too much of a parable of human handedness for comfort.

Most animals, on the other hand, developed differently because they possessed what plants did not: the power of locomotion. Because they could swim, fly, or run toward their food instead of waiting for it to come to them, they naturally evolved a mouth on the front of their body rather than on the back. As Gardner says, it was more efficient. Now front and back, as well as top and bottom, were operationally defined.

But as Gardner puts it, although land, air, and water differ as dramatically as elements can, to the animal—bird or fish alike—"its environment on the left [is] pretty much like its environment on the right."[1]

In short, its habitat is for all practical purposes symmetrical, that is to say, evenhanded in its potential for action.

For that reason, both the distance-sensing organs and ambulatory appendages of most animals—eyes and ears, feet and wings and fins—have usually evolved bilaterally, in matching, equal pairs. Thus the two sides of most animals are mirror images of each other, far more symmetrical even than lakes, mountains, or trees.

Again, however, as in the plant world, exceptions abound. The helically twisting horn of the ram, the one outsized claw of the fiddler crab, the scissorlike beak of the crossbill—each in its own distinctive way is asymmetrical.

More curious yet is the flatfish, a large family of bottom-dwellers including the sole and flounder who reach adulthood with both eyes *on the same side* (looking upward, naturally). The side may be either the left or the right, depending on which of its hundreds of sub-species you pull from the mud, and where. Some dextral soles inhabit only cold waters, some sinistral soles only warm. In every instance the difference appears to be species-specific—and unexplainable.

But the strangest of all, by far, is the anablep, an anagrammatic denizen of the deep from Latin America. A small four-eyed carp, the anablep manages to work handedness into, of all things, its sex life. Both sexes, as it happens, are either sinistral or dextral in the location of their reproductive organs. Two anableps of differing handedness simply cannot mate, which as anyone would agree is carrying handedness a bit too far. Fortunately, as Gardner sympathetically observes, the ratio is a God-given fifty-fifty; otherwise, adds Gardner, "the species would soon be in serious trouble."[2]

But these, after all, are asymmetric differences in structure, not function. If the laws of motion are truly asymmetrical at base, do we see any signs of this in how animals cope with the operationally even-handed environment around them? Do they, in brief, betray a taste for unilateral action despite the visible bilaterality of their mirror-image limbs? Are they, in a word, left-limbed or right-limbed?

Aside from the counterclockwise spiral in which bats are believed always to swarm from their caves—and the trouble trainers have teaching some horses to start a gallop with their right hoof—there is, alas, not much solid evidence to support the idea of an overriding animal preference for the left or right in any gross movement. This appears to hold experimentally up to and including mice, rats, monkeys, and the higher apes.

True, any one specimen of each may show a pronounced favoritism for either paw at the expense of the other. And like the Dewey-indoctrinated schoolboy of Depression days, they can be trained out of it. But invariably the species as a whole in any large test sample approaches random probability, the roughly fifty-fifty equilibrium of coin-flipping, with as many preferring one paw as the other, no matter what the task.

Indeed, the lack of a preference has proven so emphatic in the laboratory animals normally used for experimental extrapolations to man that animal psychologists—and some human—are beginning to use the results in arguing that handedness in people is likewise a matter of random environmental factors.

For that reason let us explore in more detail some of the more important animal findings.

Scottish shoemakers believe that the right side of hides is thicker than the left because cattle lie down on that side, legend has it. Erroneous though that has been shown by the indefatigable Richard Uhrbrock, asymmetry in animals remains an avenue of fruitful search as well as a frequent blind alley. Turning first to those most like man, in the higher apes such as gorillas, chimpanzees, orangutans, and gibbons, even-sidedness appears to be nature's dominant scheme. Either paw may be used, depending on the complexity of the task, and one or the other is often reinforced by repetition.

Clearly, environment is important, but whether it strictly determines the preference by gradually conditioning a choice that was originally random, or whether it only draws out a natural tendency dormant in the animal's organic makeup all along, is moot—at least for anthropoid apes, if not for humans.

Comparing anatomical structure only clouds the issue. In the chimpanzee and gorilla, for instance, the left upper limb weighs more; in the orangutan and gibbon it is the right upper limb. Six gorillas studied postmortem, moreover—*Australopithecus* notwithstanding—had skulls whose posterior parts were all bigger on the left, suggesting brains hemispherically differentiated in their labor.

But these physical distinctions are not very helpful because, as a species, none of these four kinds of higher apes has been shown to consistently prefer one hand or the other—or one foot, for that matter.

Monkeys and baboons, when tested experimentally, have demonstrated much the same pattern. Their hand preference is initially as weak as that of the anthropoids; and as with the anthropoids, the preference grows strong when the task is made more difficult and the animals are subjected to repeated trials (and therefore influenced by learning). What's more, under laboratory conditions monkeys show a growing preference for one foot and eye as well. Like the paw preference, it can appear on either side.

97

Curiously, their foot preference is nowhere near as common or pronounced as for the paw, although each appears on the same side in any animal that shows both. The preferred eye, in contrast, while statistically a phenomenon stronger and more common than the foot, just as frequently appears on the *opposite* side!

What exactly are we to make of this? No one knows for sure. Meanwhile, at the London zoo (writer Michael Barsley reports), the chimpanzees, grandly oblivious to the agonies of science, continue to take their afternoon tea with either or both hands, ambidextrously pouring and sipping and balancing their plates, presumably, on either knee.

Rats and mice, however—the most common experimental "stand-ins" for man because of their cheapness and the ease of surgical or chemical intervention—paradoxically differ from primates. Some rats are ambidextrous despite every effort to make them otherwise. Others are so relentlessly single-handed that after only a dozen or two reaches for food they will retain that preference for life unless disrupted by brain injury or contrary practice forced on them by the contingencies of punishment or reward.

We know that the rat's choice of hand, if it has a choice, is governed by a tiny cluster of cells housed in the cerebral hemisphere opposite the side it manifestly prefers. (In vertebrates, contralateral neural control is the rule.) Destroy that cluster with a precisely inflicted lesion and the rat will voluntarily (sic) switch to the other paw.

We know, too, that rat handedness is probably mediated by, or at least intimately related to, the presence or absence of a balance in the minute amounts of dopamine found in certain critical regions on both sides of the brain. Dopamine is one of the brain's neurotransmitters—chemicals that, as the name implies, transmit the neural impulses that govern bodily movement and sensation.

If a natural balance exists, research suggests, the rat will be ambidextrous, at least in its tendency to "rotate" (run around in circles) on the floor of its cage. If a natural balance does not exist— and researchers believe an imbalance is just as natural to rats as a balance—the rat's "scurry pattern" will be clockwise or counterclockwise, whichever direction is contralateral to the side having the higher level of dopamine. In other words, if the left side of its brain has more dopamine, the rat will rotate to the right, and vice versa.

To test whether dopamine levels have spatial significance beyond rotation, experimenters have inflicted lesions that effectively blocked the neurotransmitter's action on the handedness-controlling side of the rat's brain. Sure enough, the injured rat not only reversed the direction of its habitual rotation, it persisted in its new bias when running a T-maze, consistently taking the direction opposite its formerly entrenched tendency.

Is the initial paw preference of the single-handed rat built into it genetically or does it develop naturally—by means of what biologists and computer scientists alike would call a "positive feedback loop"—from the rat's exploratory collision with the environment? More to the point, is handedness an *effect* of the dopamine imbalance, the *cause* of it, or do both occur as the result of some other as-yet-unknown mechanism?

There can be no question that a transfer of handedness, in rats anyway, when achieved by conditioning rather than surgical intervention, involves learning. Switching hands, postmortem biochemical assays of rat brains show, inevitably results in increased production of protein—a reliable physical index to behavioral growth in rodents.

But whether that original handedness is primarily innate or learned has until recently remained an open question.

Now, however, Dr. Robert Collins, a respected animal geneticist, has come forward with a simple but extensive series of experiments to show that handedness in *mice,* at any rate, is "culturally imposed" by the directional bias or lack of it in the outside world.

To demonstrate, Collins first housed several hundred baby mice in a cage whose food container was situated exactly in the center of its front wall. Pellets could be acquired easily with either paw. In such an evenhanded environment almost half the mice were strongly right-pawed, half strongly left-pawed, and the remainder ambidextrous.

Next, Collins put some 300 more baby mice into cages which were engineered to produce a bias. Half had to eat from containers on the extreme right side of the front wall, half from containers on the extreme left. As Collins's environmental thesis predicted, in the right-biased cage the mice were overwhelmingly right-handed, in the left-biased cage the opposite. Most significant of all to Collins, those who stubbornly resisted either bias made up 8 and 14 percent of the two populations respectively, or *about the same as left-handers in the right-leaning world of human beings.*

His findings, however, failed to explain why these dozens of anomalous rats should persist with their maverick style of eating in the face of pellet dispensers expressly designed to make eating such an awkward chore for the nonconformist. Perhaps, driven by their disparate dopamine levels, they were just born troublemakers, misfits, renegades—as some theorists have been moved to explain similarly uncooperative humans.

Emboldened by his success, Collins then was prompted to ask, "If right- and left-handedness in mice are not attributable to genetic influences, are these forms also non-genetic in humans?"[3]

It was, and is, an enduringly good question. But when Collins sought to extend his own particular train of argument to man, he ran headlong into stiff resistance from other scientists already there. Assailing his use of statistics as erroneous, futile, and inconsistent, they dismissed his theoretical model of mouse-as-man as "a tautology"[4] (needless redundancy).

"Although Collins is very likely correct in concluding that paw preference in mice is without genetic basis," they concluded in a paragon of scientific understatement, "the mouse, unfortunately, is not always a prototype for man."[5]

Nor, for that matter, is the anthropoid ape or the monkey—in a far more obvious way than brain structure. Man differs, as we shall now see, in yet another striking way that one researcher believes could have a lot to do with asymmetry in the laws of motion—and ultimately, human handedness.

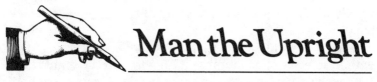 # Man the Upright

9

Into this apparently-ambidextrous-but-at-base-curiously-left-handed material world walked man. Other animals, as we have seen, were structurally affected by the demands of their environment, but only in a generally evenhanded way. Never, in any way we can detect, has nature forced them, as a species, away from overall randomness in their use of one side or the other.

Man, however, is unique. He has many names that celebrate that uniqueness: *homo sapiens,* the thinker, *homo faber,* the maker, *homo ludens,* the player. But from the standpoint of handedness, the most useful may well be *homo erectus,* upright man—for a deceptively simple reason that at least one researcher is convinced may have the farthest-reaching ramifications.

As the distinguished Boston neurophysiologist Paul Yakovlev has long pointed out, man alone among animals stands solely on his own two feet, resolutely at right angles to his environment. As a consequence only he, according to Yakovlev's arresting theory, occupies space as a "second-class lever" with the awesome power of an Archimedes to "move the world"[1] off its hinges, metaphorically speaking.

That he has done so with his thought, his tools, even his play, can readily be seen in such diverse human products as the theory of relativity, the internal combustion engine, and the Super Bowl. But what has any of this to do with which hand he favors?

Yakovlev would argue that it has almost everything to do with it, in a sense as literal as it is figurative. To understand the mechanical sense, however, it becomes necessary both to know what a second-class lever is and to visualize how the principle still applies when, in effect, it is stood on end as the ultimate "open action system"[2] that man is.

To begin with, there are three basic classes of levers in mechanics. These hold for the most sophisticated and supple muscular processes as well as for the simplest, crudest, most rigid machine relationships.

In the first-class lever, the *fulcrum,* or point of support, is between the mover and the moved. A seasaw—when it sees or saws—is a first-class lever (Figure 5A). In the second-class lever, *the thing to be moved* is between the mover and the fulcrum. A good example is the wheelbarrow (Figure 5B). In the third-class lever, the *mover* is between the fulcrum and the thing to be moved. Its action is invoked whenever you shut a door by giving it a push near the hinge (Figure 5C).

Organically speaking, Yakovlev contends, all forms of vertebrate life up through the lower primates are limited to horizontally-based first- and third-class levers in their movements (figures 6A, 6B, and 6C). This is true, he says,

104

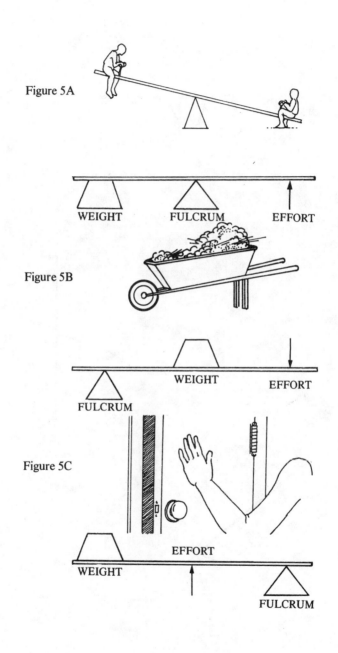

Figure 5A

WEIGHT   FULCRUM   EFFORT

Figure 5B

WEIGHT   EFFORT

FULCRUM

Figure 5C

WEIGHT   EFFORT

FULCRUM

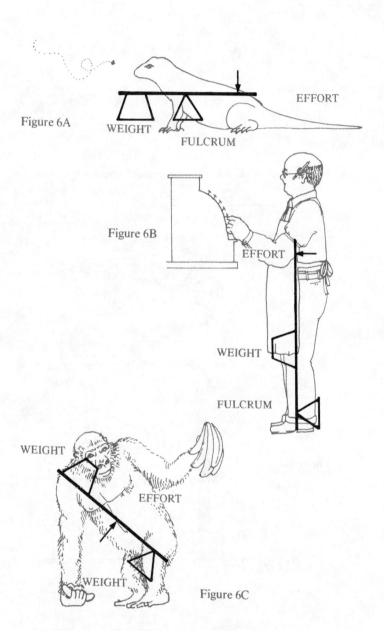

Figure 6A

EFFORT

WEIGHT

FULCRUM

Figure 6B

EFFORT

WEIGHT

FULCRUM

WEIGHT

EFFORT

WEIGHT

Figure 6C

because they live more or less parallel to the plane of gravity's pull and lack the fulcrum of an upright second-class lever that would lift their efforts free of the body contours that bind them. Just imagine, if you will, a lizard trying to operate a cash register or an oyster driving a bus. Neither has a second-class lever to its name. Only man unreservedly does. (Even the higher primates are reduced to walking on their knuckles part of the time.)

This unique ability to operate on outside space at right angles to the body's unrelenting upright axis Yakovlev sees as crucial to man's dominion. He achieves it by simply (simply!) planting his feet in the earth, squarely facing the natural forces arrayed against him, and dynamically getting on with the job of molding the world in his own image as the planet's prime mover-and-shaker.

This he does, Yakovlev would have it, through both the manufacture and manipulation (words significantly rooted in the Latin word for *hand*) of tools, of instruments for measure and counting, of ideas. These acts in turn, Yakovlev argues, convert man's excess internal energy into work that transforms the external world around him. Thus *by his own hand* does he impress himself indelibly on nature.

But the question persists. Why does he do this with one hand or the other, preferably one, the right, and rarely both or either interchangeably?

Simple, really—or so says Yakovlev. Contrary to the physicist's world view, he argues, the external environment of natural space has none of our human sense of absolute symmetry to shape it. Any hint of evenhandedness, we put there. Apart from the mountain's accidental reflection in the lake, it has no mirror image of an antithetical existence.

At the molecular level and below, the matter *in it* certainly has such mirror images, as we have seen and Yakovlev recognizes. But as a totality, as an all-enveloping operational whole, external space has not. Man-made structures aside, external space in its overall macroscopic form—as defined by the great jumble of gross natural matter in it—appears uneven, randomly dispersed, empty of any change and motion that are equally balanced directionally.

It is this fact, Yakovlev believes, that profoundly determines our choice of hand.

As he explains it, any object or event we deal with in the external world differs from all others in both position and what he calls its "velocity of motion."[3] Put with idiot simplicity, no two occupy the same physical space at any given instant. Consequently no one relates to, or behaves in, space exactly like another. What could be more obvious?

Its "rightness" or "leftness," however, exists not in the thing itself or in the space it occupies. It exists, rather, in the thing's *spatial relationship to us as we are conscious of it.*

In other words, if we are facing each other, what is on the right or the left of me hasn't the same meaning for you. Its meaning, in fact, is exactly reversed in each consciousness. If we are talking to each other on the telephone, furthermore, left and right have *no concrete meaning at all* in the absence of a common reference point. They exist only abstractly. But there, in the abstract, the concepts are overlayed operationally with our built-in sense of symmetry, and literally mirrored in our mind.

That consciousness, moreover, Yakovlev goes on, is moored to the world's wider reality by three coordinates of existence: space, time, and a lifelong awareness of our bodily self. Whenever we relate to an external object or event, he would have it, these coordinates are called into play. It is they which enable us to anchor the object or event in physical reality by "plotting" its spatial relation to us on the vibrant grid of our consciousness.

Now, our prime levers of bodily action are the hands, continues Yakovlev. Hands are bilateral, as we know, and for practical purposes organically symmetrical by nature. If external space were likewise equally divisible and apprehendable as such, Yakovlev thinks, man would indeed be uniformly ambidextrous in his "handling" of it.

But no, he insists, external space is actually dissymmetric, skewed, warped—to one side. As a result, he says, economy and efficiency demand that our manual use of it preferentially attract one hand at the expense of the other, although the lesser hand remains usable.

In fact, the curious diagonal relationship mentioned earlier that most often exists between the controlling left hemisphere of our brain and the right hand, Yakovlev sees as one faithfully reflecting, mirror-fashion, the outside space in which we live. As a species we are biased to our right, he claims, just as—and *because*—space is biased to its left.

As we have seen, opposite-side neural control of the body by the brain is found in the ambidextrous higher apes as well. What makes man different is his expression of a *preference*, which gives his manual movements in space both a *torque* (or twist) and a *skew* (or slant). It is this torque and this slant, Yakovlev believes, that are dictated by the mirror torque of space together with the hand's changing orientation or line of skew in space. The key of the hand, as it were, is ground to fit the lock of space, and only upright man has (or even needs, for his work) that key.

The image of man groping around in outright *nothingness* for a more-than-metaphorical handle on things—like some drunk blundering through the midnight darkness for the right door—does not rest easy on the mind. Where, we must ask, is Yakovlev's proof that space itself has a natural torque? We know a world of things exists smaller than the eye, or even the microscope, can see. But space is not a *thing*. Space is the *absence* of things. Isn't it?

Physicists asked themselves the same astonishing question when the reassuring edifice that parity had been crumbled and fell in about their heads. As Martin Gardner writes:

> Could space itself possess, at every point, some sort of intrinsic handedness? Both the classical physics of Newton and the equations of modern relativity theory and quantum theory assume that space is completely isotropic. This means that one direction in space is no different from another; space is spherically symmetrical. Is it possible to construct models of the cosmos in which space has an intrinsic handedness?[4]

Yes, Gardner found in examining the infamous weak interactions of the K-meson, mathematicians could. Or at least they could make mathematical models of such a space, though the trick was far from simple even in theory: "The twist has to be present at every point . . . [Also] one has to construct a space in which there is some sort of fine, unobservable 'grain' which provides a uniform asymmetric twist . . ."[5]

Given those conditions, Gardner reported, weak interactions could violate parity as "a slow-moving ball . . . or a ball as small as a pea"[6] would be guided in its path by a warp in a bowling alley too subtle to be seen. Either projectile would hook right or left, depending on the alley's direction of skew (and perhaps the torque you imparted to the ball on releasing it?).

Given stronger forces, however—and here Gardner's thoughts move speedily away from Yakovlev's with no impeding grain evident in his argument—"the subtle, minute twist of space would be negligible,"[7] much as it would be on the warped bowling lane if, as bowlers often do, you detected the skew and overcame it by releasing the ball more powerfully.

Gardner, then, holds no brief for a torque in space—even if physicist Eugene Wigner, by extension of his speculations on the shifting laws of motion, might appear to hold out such a farfetched possibility at least in theory.

One of Yakovlev's colleagues in the field of handedness research is not so charitable. Jerre Levy calls the entire argument "sheer mysticism." There is, she says, "absolutely no evidence of any rightward torque to space. Quite possibly, [he] believes that the overthrow of parity conservation in elementary particle physics implies this. It does no such thing."[8]

Levy, like most scientists, subscribes to the accepted view that living proteins are left-handed due to "pure chance"[9] and not to some mysterious force in either space or motion that continues to shape our predominant preference for the right hand. "It is true that our biological organisms are built out of [left-handed] amino acids. But that fact should have nothing to do with it, because the only thing that the genes are doing is building proteins.

"Those proteins—every single one is an optical isomer that will either rotate polarized light to the left or to the right. Even had we been built out of dextro-amino acids, their tertiary structures—the complex, folded-up shapes— could have been exactly as they are now. The primary structure of a protein is really irrelevant in terms of biological activity. Even the secondary structure is irrelevant."[10]

In any case, Levy adds, "quantum mechanical events have never played, do not play, and can never play any role in biological evolution.

"We evolved, and continue to do so, in accordance with purely Newtonian forces."[11]

Undaunted, Yakovlev reiterates that it is "a challenging and as yet unexplained fact"[12] that "random, ever-changing, and unpredictable forces"[13] render external space "wide open [boundless] and *dissymmetrical*"[14] in the Pasteurian sense. It is *space* that is *skewed to the left,* not man to the right, he stoutly maintains, although man in addressing himself and his work to this permeating skew must do so with an answering right-handed torque:

> This, the "majority" side, inexorably enough, is called the "right" side, and the bias of the . . . torque is reflected in all products (artifacts) of human thought, language and manufacture.[15]

When challenged to support his notion of a torque in space, Yakovlev calls the fact of its existence "empirical,"[16] although others might—and do—call it wishful thinking, particularly on the basis of published remarks such as these:

> There must be some "forces" that turn the torque . . . in 80 percent of mankind to one and the same side . . . I assume that these . . . are forces *external* to the body. I assume that the turn of the torque and the sense of bias in the skew to this—the "majority" side—must be more economical in energy consumed in work.[17]

Even then, the archeological evidence reviewed earlier forces Yakovlev to concede that in the life of early man, things were different.

"Evidently within the past hundred thousand years or less," he says, "either the 'screw' which propels human action . . . has become threaded differently or the structure of physical space itself has changed."[18]

Having faced himself with such a Solomonlike choice over a decade ago in a major speech before the national Society of Biological Psychiatry, Yakovlev still managed to surprise with his selection:

"We live," he told the audience, "in a 'right-handed' . . . non-symmetrical, lopsided world."[19]

Appealing though such an esoteric idea may be—to left-handers, anyway—the underlying simile of the lock-and-key has an open-ended quality that instantly raises up the issue it has just buried. It is too much like the chicken and the egg for comfort. Which came first? Was the key ground to fit the lock or was the lock molded to fit the key?

Without either, the other simply won't work. Man—the upright thinker, maker, player—surely shapes space, as Yakovlev would be the first to admit. But space as an envelope to live in shapes man just as surely. Modifying an analogy from neuroscientist Donald Hebb of Canada, to question whether the torque was initially in man or in the world around him—much less where it might be today—makes about as much sense as asking which most determines the area of a field, its length or width?

A better question would be, How is physical man himself organized as an entity to reflect or express this natural torque, wherever it began and if it exists? What is its wellspring, its secret source, within us?

Paradoxically, it is here Levy and Yakovlev find common ground—and we a measure of much-needed illumination.

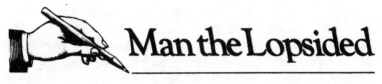

Man the Lopsided

10

To the naked eye, physical man appears the very soul of symmetry. His eyes, ears, arms, hands, breasts, legs, and feet are neatly lateralized to either side of his body. His nose, mouth, buttocks, and sex organs are elegantly divided down the middle. His sides, in short, neatly mirror-image each other. Superficially viewed, not even Zeus, once his godly temper cooled, would find his modified creation structurally unworthy of Olympus, as observers of any beauty or body-building contest would quickly agree.

But pleasingly regular though it may strike our sight, even this symmetrical alignment is more apparent than real. As any tailor and glove-maker can tell you, one leg and arm are longer, one hand bigger, because our habits of stance and use tend to favor one side's development over the other. Less apparent but just as real is a phenomenon like *trichogyria*, the whorl of every hair on our heads, which is basically clockwise in right-handers, counterclockwise in left. What's more, in males, to lessen the skin contact that can generate sperm-killing heat, nature has conveniently arranged for one testicle to hang lower. (According to one study, it is usually on the side opposite the hand we prefer for most tasks.)

What natural symmetry that remains goes hardly more than skin-deep. Lungs, kidneys, and ovaries are spatially balanced in offsetting pairs, but other vital organs such as the heart, the pancreas, the stomach, and the liver contribute nothing to the notion of human symmetry—either apart or, in terms of ensuring a balanced body weight, together. In fact, they obliterate it. The stomach, heart, and pancreas are on the left, the liver is on the right. The twists and turns of our intestines likewise obey no laws of natural equity. Even one of our lungs—usually the right—is larger than the other.

But can such natural disparities be dismissed as unimportant or held up as crucial to hand perference? That's the question. As it happens, such a lopsided visceral distribution gave rise to one of the earliest theories grounded in the physical nature of man. Called the mechanical theory, it argued—without help from Yakovlev—that since the greater weight of the liver and lungs lay in the right half of the body, man tended to balance better on his left foot, which freed his right hand to act more effectively.

Gravity was displaced to the right, supporters of the mechanical theory maintained, as much as three-tenths of an inch. The muscles on that side, therefore, were better developed. From that came the initial superiority of function upon which the full weight of society's historic bias could be erected, with no embarrassing loss of balance in logic.

Such a theory might hold, of course, until one simple, two-pronged question was asked:

Why were the higher apes ambidextrous, when their viscera were all but identically arrayed to man's? And how, then, explain the pesky southpaw, unless his organs bulked decidedly to port, a phenomenon found only in one of a pair of Siamese twins, or in the anomalous single birth accompanied usually by congenital defects? (*Southpaw*, by the way, was coined by a Chicago sportswriter to describe left-handed pitchers who, in an old ballpark there, faced south when they went into their stretch with a runner on first.)

Mirror-image reversals of handedness are, in fact, pronounced in Siamese twins, those identical infants left locked together fetally in some manner when the single egg that produces them fails to divide normally. That is, one will be right-handed, the other left. But such accidents of nature as the Siamese are far too rare to tell us anything much about the norm.

As for the statistically more frequent single births with inverted viscera—heart on the right, say, liver on the left—left-handedness is no more common to them than to the population as a whole.

These same exceptions—left-handed people and ambidextrous primates—appear equally to demolish as possible sources of hand preference such surprising organic asymmetries as the normally unequal flow and pressure of arterial blood on either side of our body. Again, it is the right that is favored. And again, the left-hander and the ape do not differ physically from the right-handed in any fundamental way.

Purely mechanical and physical theories, in sum, simply do not wash.

Only when we get to the way in which his nervous system is wired do we begin to perceive, as cyberneticist Norman Dalkey so aptly puts it in another context, differences that not only exist, but "that make a difference."[1] It is here that

Yakovlev and Levy, as we shall see later, agree on something of vital significance.

Postmortem dissection, in fetuses and newborns, of the lower brain and upper spinal cord, Yakovlev and his associate Pasko Rakic report, exposes a "wiring diagram" that offers persuasive evidence for a naturally dominant side in at least some of our movements. Generally, they found, nerves leading from the left cerebral hemisphere to the right half of the neck are not only woven to "have the right-of-way,"[2] there are more of them. On the right there are also more of the relatively fewer nerves that connect the same side of the brain and body. In short, the right in most cases appears to get more neural "juice"—in the neck, anyway.

(These fibers, curiously enough, are as helical, as screwlike, in their twistings as any morning glory or bindweed. Is man their brother? Does biology recapitulate botany?)

Whether this dextral right-of-way is true of the hand, not to mention the entire body, must await a large-scale, tedious dissection of totally intact spinal cords if we want direct proof. The statistical picture is intriguing: 87 percent of the specimens showed right-side neural preponderance and 13 did not—which fits remarkably with handedness discrimination when all of the major studies are averaged, varied though their results and approaches may be.

But statistics, we know, can be misleading. And in this instance, the neatness of the proportional fit to handedness does appear accidental. For according to clinical records, only *four* of the postmortem subjects had been left-handed —and none of them at all were in the 13 percent where they might have been expected to be. On the contrary, their preponderances of nerves were woven left-to-right, or *exactly opposite* what would have been predicted were handedness directly and indisputably linked to neural right-of-way.

It was this crucial discrepancy that led Yakovlev to back away from the brain-body "wiring plan" as the ultimate cause of human hand preference and to cast his lot with an unseen torque in space—although he still considers the "right-handed management"[3] of that torque to be more "economical of the visceral energy of the human body"[4] because of its usual preponderance of left-to-right neural fibers. Levy, as we will learn, makes a different but related use of this data in espousing an exciting new concept.

At any rate, one thing is clear: Postmortem speculation is one thing, an established and meaningful connection with the living body is quite another. As late as a decade ago we thought motor preference of the most elemental sort did not get wired in before we were seven or eight. A preferred side for sensory perception, we thought, did not develop until twice that age. Indeed, that electrical activity in the brain of an infant had any meaning at all—outside of injury—was unheard of.

Now, however, thanks to recent developments in electroencephalograph technology (EEG), new if indirect evidence has been unearthed to show that the biased neural "wiring" Yakovlev and Rakic found anatomically does have definite functional significance. Infants in their first hours, for instance, exhibit distinctively different electrical activity in each of their cerebral hemispheres. Not only that, but one side of the brain, usually the left, is more active.

Then, too, consider the common "tonic reflex" of the newborn, that familiar stretching movement in which it extends in the direction it faces the arms, legs, hands, and feet on that side, while flexing those opposite. *A preferred direction* in such extension, new research makes clear, occurs during the first two months after birth. And although it usually vanishes after five months, in three-quarters of the infants tested that preference proved a tip-off as to *which hand they would eventually come to prefer.*

Nor is such an indirect neurological indicator limited to neck movements in infancy—or to pure motor phenomena. As early as our second day of life, researchers have determined, we express a distinct preference for one side or the other, both in the direction we turn our head and in our sensitivity to stimuli.

In general, they write, "the newborn infant spends the overwhelming majority of his time with his head turned to the right,"[5] as might be expected. In addition, it responds to sound, sight, and facial touch better on that side, too. Furthermore, when a team of Czech neurologists examined the cerebral hemispheres with an EEG to see which side of the brain reacted most to a small shock given both hands, it was *the side controlling the preferred hand* that registered the higher amplitides. In other words, in all but a few cases the left half of the brain was more sensitive in the right-hander, the right half in the left-hander.

Indeed, varied experiments by different researchers on subjects of all ages now suggest in general that such a pronounced sidedness may well apply to *all* the body's sensorimotor nerves *throughout* life. In plain words, we do appear to be neurologically lopsided, and usually to the right. We do appear, in brief, to be *wired* that way, favoring one side or the other, and no mistake.

Unfortunately, however, none of these many tests are all that helpful in clinically establishing preferred handedness, much less in explaining it. Why? Because the relationship of neurological sidedness to hand use is anything but the model of clarity and consistency we would like. For example, in a caliper study of touch sensitivity on the lips, tongue, and fingertips of college students, one side was consistently more sensitive than the other. But no directional trend was evident—for either right-handers or left-handers.

In maddening contrast, two other adult groups tested on differing tactile measures—pain and the skin's electrical potential—demonstrated a strong skew to the right—*regardless* of their hand preference. Not only did one mixed group subjectively feel the pain of dunking their right hands in unbearably icy water more than their left. The other group, when bombarded with loud sounds, flashes of bright light, and minute shocks to the hands, wrists, and little fingers, registered skin responses that were much higher on the right side of their bodies. Preferred hand be damned.

Strangely enough, although recording the skin's electrical potential smacks impressively of scientific objectivity, the researchers felt its subtle susceptibility to emotional contamination might have been the very thing that spoiled the positive relationship they fully expected to find between the preferred hand and the higher reading.

As we know, our skin is, in physiologist Barbara Brown's words, a "bright mirror of our emotions."[6] We have only to feel it "crawl" at the sight or thought of something revolting to know the practical truth of this. Although right-handed subjects were a cinch to find, the experimenters reported, left-handers took several months to round up in sufficient numbers. As a result, they were greeted with such enthusiasm their skins may have gotten a "glow on" that fouled the normal potentials on which these studies must be based, involving as they do recording and analyzing divergences from such a baseline.

Under these circumstances, then, what are we to make of a squeeze test in which both left-handers and right-handers show a stronger "readiness" electrically in the brain's left hemisphere when the right hand it controls is prepared to grip—but only the right-hander does when the situation is reversed? One might reasonably expect the left-hander to shine when ready to exhibit his manual preference, but no, his readiness to perform proves inferior, further confounding the lines of experimental evidence.

Perhaps the most exasperating instance of the left-hander's innate refusal to be neatly pinned down by neurology lies in the related phenomenon of eyedness. We know that people not only prefer one eye to the other when asked to demonstrate a choice between the two, but unconsciously betray a bent for that eye in visual tasks where both appear to be operating together.

For example, ask yourself which eye you use when aiming a rifle, peering through a telescope, or peeping through a keyhole. The chances are overwhelming that this same eye will prove to be the one that leads the other when reading, according to painstaking slow-motion videotape studies of the eyes' ballistic movements across the printed page. Like the first of a pair of perfectly matched horses harnessed tandem fashion, it pulls and guides the other as they nimbly leap through their traces.

Simpler yet, test your own sighting preference by holding a pencil or pen upright in front of your eyes and masking with it one of the vertical lines of the door or window in the opposite wall.

Now close your left eye. Is the line still covered or not? If it is, you normally sight with your right eye. Closing the left eye makes no difference. But if it is not still covered, you normally sight with your left eye, a fact which can be speedily proven by merely closing your right eye instead and watching what happens. The line stays masked because the right eye is superfluous.

How nice and tidy it would be if I. A. Porta had been right way back in 1593:

> Nature has bestowed on us eyes in pairs, one at the right hand and one at the left, so that if we are to see anything at the right hand we make use of the right eye . . .[7]

Such an assumed direct link between same-side eye and hand would suggest, of course, that those who preferred the right would do so both manually and visually, the same for the left. If you were right-handed you would be right-eyed, if you were left-handed, left-eyed. Correct?

Indeed, one major study found that more than eight out of ten people tested by such a simple objective method as pencil-sighting were right-eyed—roughly the same proportion as that usually found for right-hand preference. Unfortunately, a closer look at the data from another viewpoint blows such an elegant statistical mesh sky-high. Of the right-eyed only three out of four were right-handed in all eleven tasks of a manual test. The test data were shamelessly mixed.

Typically, there were too few who were left-handed in all eleven tasks to permit any kind of meaningful comparison.

Taken all together, however, this experiment and other large-scale studies indicate that while those living perversities, the left-handers, are just as likely to favor one eye as the other, right-handers at least lean to right-eyedness to a degree exceeding pure chance. Any inference that cause-and-effect might be operating here is undercut by the simple fact that the congenitally blind demonstrate about the same proportion of hand preference as people who can see.

All in all, researchers have felt safe in concluding only that in right-handers there is an underlying *correlation* with eyedness: a common influence from a third source, say, the lopsided neural organization Yakovlev and Rakic exposed in microcosm.

Even there, the neural structure of our eyes becomes so complicated it all but annihilates handy generalization. Only the *movements* of either eye are crisply controlled by the opposite side of the brain. Visual perception, to make matters appallingly worse, is vertically divided in both eyes. All that is seen to the *right* of an invisible midline in each eye is sent to the *left* hemisphere, all that is seen to the *left* of that invisible midline in each eye is sent to the *right* hemisphere.

The split in our vision, of which we are acutely unaware, is further confounded by the fact that our cerebral hemispheres are not mirror images of each other in function, either.

Can it be that all this is related? Perhaps in the end only our lopsided brain knows for sure—a monumental possibility we will now examine.

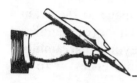# Our
Uneven Brain

11

If by magic you could peer into the living human brain and watch it transparently in action, you would see nothing to remotely suggest the enticing neurological truth that may set man and his handedness forever apart from all other animals and theirs: In its operation, his brain alone appears to be fully asymmetrical.

Perched on top of the brain stem and limbic lobe in front of the cerebellum, the two halves of our cerebrum sit like the matching meats of the walnut, connected by bands of neural tissue called commissures. To casual inspection these moist folded hemispheres of pinkish grey jelly are mirror images of each other. Anatomically, however, postmortem dissection has shown a small but significant difference: a slight elongation in the left temple area of most specimens where our capacity for expressive language is known to be generally localized.

Under the electron microscope's mullionfold magnification, furthermore, the neurons, or nerve cells, of the left hemisphere have typically revealed what brain injuries have for generations led us to suspect: that it has more precise point-to-point pathways than the more diffuse nerve arrangement of the right hemisphere.

For that reason, damage to the left side of the brain usually results in more specific loss of limb movement, right-side senses, or the ability to talk. Damage to the brain's right hemisphere, in contrast, results in a more generalized impairment of the body's left half. Beyond that, until recent years these subtle anatomical differences were not thought to be especially meaningful.

Now, however, thanks to prolonged experimental study and decades of clinical observation, we are discovering, to our growing amazement, that these structural distinctions underlie dramatically contrasting brain functions and organization. In sum, the two hemispheres are only rough mirror images *outwardly*. Inside, neurally speaking, they are as different in the way they are "wired" as they can be. They differ so much functionally, in fact, that many respected researchers have taken to calling them our "two brains."

One of these dual "brains"—usually our left hemisphere, we have learned—contains our capacity not only for generating language but for making and manipulating the symbols of higher mathematics. As a consequence, it tends in its thinking to be linear (like language) and analytic (like math) as well as logical, abstract, and conceptual (like both symbol-using systems). It pays attention to details rather than form, to parts instead of the whole, to the trees and not the forest.

The "brain" most often housed in our right hemisphere,

by contrast, is home to a subtle and not-entirely-understood array of visual and spatial abilities having as their common bond the fusing, reevoking, and synthesizing of perceptual images—primarily those of sight, sound, and touch. These imagistic attributes, of course, are embodied in what we customarily think of as art: painting, sculpture, dance, music, theater.

But we are beginning to suspect that they also inform such oblique kinds of intellect as intuition and insight, hunches and "gut feelings," the holistic grasping of "the big picture" from the fragmentary pieces of an incomplete puzzle posed by many kinds of problem solving we frequently confront in life.

The right hemisphere, moreover, is simultaneous in its function, not sequential; concrete, not abstract. It compares configurations, not concepts.

All in all, as Jerre Levy eloquently puts it, the current state of brain research suggests that

> . . . the human cerebral hemispheres exist in a symbiotic relationship in which both the capacities and motivations to act are complementary. Each side of the brain is able to perform and chooses to perform a certain set of cognitive tasks which the other side finds difficult or distasteful or both. . . . The right hemisphere synthesizes over space. The left hemisphere analyzes over time. . . . The right hemisphere codes sensory input in terms of images, the left hemisphere in terms of linguistic descriptions. The right hemisphere lacks an . . . analyzer; the left hemisphere lacks a . . . pattern synthesizer.[1]

Whether our two brains alternate in their response to the environment—one resting and the other working, depending on the nature of the stimulus—or whether they function simultaneously—each processing out of the total situation those facets it does best—remains one of the more intriguing questions facing neuroscience.

So does the ticklish issue of which hemisphere exercises "executive control" of what we have come to consider our unitary consciousness. Who, in a word, is in charge?

Tentatively it has been suggested that the ego, or self-consciousness, resides in the left hemisphere with the language that gives it expression, while the outward, or environmental, consciousness resides in the right hemisphere with the perceptions that reflect it.

Paradoxically, neurosurgeon Joseph Bogen theorizes, the left hemisphere sees the person existing in the world, the right hemisphere sees the world existing in the person. But neither concept alone would seem fully to capture what Bogen calls "the inner conviction of Oneness [that] is the most cherished opinion of Western man."[2]

One thing we increasingly suspect, however, as the result of highly sensitive measures that enable us to test each hemisphere of the normal, intact brain separately: *contralateral control is the rule*, in human information processing, too, just as in the vastly simpler realms of sensory and motor function.

Which is to say that, in general, the senses, limbs, *and* intellectual operations of either side are primarily tied to the opposite side of the brain. In other words, just as the left hemisphere in most people moves the right arm and leg and is sensitive to pain in that hand and foot, so does it appear to impress its mode of cerebration on that side.

The converse appears equally true of the right hemisphere and the left side of the body. For example, the *right* ear is better at processing language than the left because it "reports" to the linguistically superior left hemisphere. But

128

the *left* hand is better at reading Braille because it reports to a right hemisphere whose spatial intelligence makes it far more sensitive to such tactile patterns.

All this is relative, of course. In the intact brain the commissures routinely transmit nerve impulses between the hemispheres, insuring the kind of swift and constant communication that guarantees a comparable caliber of performance on *any* mental task by either side of the body. But cut the commissures and the two halves of the brain are dramatically divided against each other, not only in their contrasting mental abilities, but in their sensorimotor discriminations as well.

In a series of last-ditch operations to stop the spread of otherwise intractible epilepsy across the commissures, patient after patient has demonstrated conclusively that in both perception and expression his mind has been rendered schizophrenic: literally split in two. Destroy the bridges across which the two hemispheres normally exchange information, ingenious and careful "solo" tests of each hemisphere have showed, and you destroy the access of each to the gifts of the other.

Neither hemisphere knows what the other has seen, heard, or touched with "its side" of the body. (Smell and taste, relying as they do on a single shared organ, are too unified for such dual discriminations.) Even more astonishing, not only does each hemisphere fall down when called upon to solve experimental problems the other is better at, both are so intent on protecting their own intellectual turf that they sometimes wrest control of the opposite side of the body away from the other hemisphere on tasks where they shine. At such times they are like spoiled children; at other times they might as well be walking around in different bodies.

Normally such a split is not nearly so pronounced, of course. Delays connoting a telltale transfer from one hemisphere (that dislikes a task) to the other (that dotes on it) are smoothly synchronized, detectable and measurable only on a split-second basis. But the division of labor—and consequent difference in brain organization—are there, despite the mind's masquerade as a plausible whole.

That raises a further fascinating question. Consciousness aside, some researchers feel the two hemispheres actually *compete* to determine our overriding style of cognition in life. They believe that we tend to favor the functions of one hemisphere or the other in our mental behavior—that as thinkers we are apt to be either verbal-and-symbolic or perceptive-and-imagistic.

At its most sublime, such a disparity, when coupled to exceptional talent, can lead to a Shakespeare or a Michelangelo. At its more mundane, perhaps, emphasizing the one kind of brain organization produces a person who sweeps the *floor,* while emphasizing the other produces a person who sweeps the *dirt.*

If so, is this somehow significantly related to our preference for one hand at the expense of the other, motor-controlled as each hand is by the opposite hemisphere?

Tempting as such parallels are, the answer is not that simple. Contralateral neural control is an all-emcompassing if not simple fact of vertebrate life, one that traces back through evolution to the most primitive spinal reflex of the flattened marine organism known as the lancelet or amphioxus.

As Levy describes its humble beginnings, "our moronic protovertebrate ancestors had no distance receptors, lay buried in the sand and filter-fed, and had only one striated muscle response: a coiling reflex *away* from the source of a stimulus.

"Thus, a stimulus on the left produced muscle contraction on the right. Because the stupid beast had *no* approach reflexes, everything was crossed and all its descendants inherited it"—including man.[3]

Even lesser animals today demonstrate not only such neural cross-connections but signs of at least a primitive asymmetry in their nervous systems. An "imbalance in dopamine levels," after all, is just another way of saying that rats have a hemispheric asymmetry in their brain chemistry. What's more, other experiments have indicated that cats, monkeys, and baboons often perform and learn far better in one hemisphere than the other (when the two are surgically separated), depending on whether the task is visual or tactile. Finally, monkeys and baboons exhibit a decided imbalance in the distribution of spinal-cord fibers similar to that of man—although they, like all the other animals mentioned, fail to show the hand preference that would make such a connection promising.

Such asymmetries in the brain and nervous system of man are, of course, much more profound and pervasive in their expression, as befits his vastly greater neural complexity. When confronted with numerical tasks tailored to his abstract hemisphere, for example, man consistently shows by his EEG readings a surge of electricity on that side of the brain, indicating that it is "switched on," ready to go, vibrantly expectant.

More dramatic yet, he visibly betrays his brain's bilateralization of language and spatial skills, as well as the onset of either activity, simply by the way he moves his eyes. Asked to stare straight ahead, he does so by directing both

131

hemispheres to fix their attention—the focus of the visual half-fields each controls—forward. This forced balance, however, is disrupted when either hemisphere is asked to solve a problem demanding its special competence. The competing stimulus, psychologist Marcel Kinsbourne believes, in effect "overloads" the already activated hemisphere, driving the balance of attention off-center and, given the pull of the opposing hemisphere, in the opposite direction. Thus, given a verbal problem, our eyes roll right; given a spatial problem, they roll left.

But neither cerebral condition—opposite-side neural control and asymmetry of hemispheric function—together or alone explain man's unique handedness. Can it be, then, that there *is* no connection? Hardly. Psychologists at Tel Aviv University have found that electrical resistance in the skin of either hand goes up or down depending on the nature of the task it is given—as might be predicted, in right-handers the right hand on verbal and numerical tasks, the left hand on visual-imagery tasks. So a strong connection does exist. Exactly what is it?

We don't know, but neurophysiology today has come a long way from the simple cause-and-effect assumption popular a century ago, when neurologists, noting that language lay on the left side in over 90 percent of the brain-damaged cases studied for aphasia (loss of speech), decided to give our symbol-making abilities all the better of it. They concluded, in the words of Paul Broca, that "we are right-handed because we are left-brained."[4]

Some time after that, an antithetical critic chimed in with a thesis that turned things around completely. "We are left-brained," he said, "because we are right-handed."[5]

Neither explanation, we have since learned, can really be true. If they were, most English teachers and certified public accountants would be right-handed, and most painters and sculptors left-handed. Indeed, we now know, six out of ten left-handers have their language centers on the *left* side, not on the right, as the doctrine of contralateral neural control would lead us to expect.

(To complicate matters even more, some left-handers, we know from converging lines of clinical and experimental research, have language on *both* sides of their brain.)

This curious same-sidedness (and double-sidedness) prompted Broca's successors to dismiss any serious connection between handedness and brain organization for the next hundred years. Only recently, on the strength of exciting new evidence, has the idea been renewed—as we will see in the concluding chapter.

Finally, in passing, what are we—what is anyone—to make of the startling claim by devotees of French obstetrician Frederick Leboyer that his controversial technique of *Birth Without Violence* results in babies who *exhibit no manual preference,* who are *uniformly adroit with either hand?*

Leboyer babies are delivered in shadow with a soothing bath and massage, not jerked into consciousness with the "fantastic aggression"[6] of bright lights and a spine-twisting spank on the butt while suspended upside down in the terrifying void of space. According to preliminary reports from a long-term follow-up study, they grow to be alert, relaxed, peaceful, inventive children who "use both their hands well."[7]

Clinical psychologist Danielle Rapoport steadfastly refuses to comment at this early stage of the investigation of their alleged lack of handedness. But the implication of such a development, if true, would be a decided bombshell to most of the cherished notions about the importance of nervous-system laterality. It would say nothing less than this: Ambidexterity is one of the bountiful and beneficent effects of a tranquil penumbrous birth. Ergo, preferred handedness is one of the most traumatic consequences of obstetrics as traditionally practiced.

Understandably, advocates of a genetic base to handedness are reluctant to entertain such an idea. But then, they have their hands full already, as we shall now see.

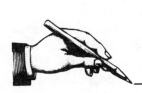

Heredity, Environment, or Insult?

12

How do we know left from right?

The question is not as simpleminded as it seems. We do it, as the old joke goes, the way porcupines make love: with great difficulty. For as we have seen, unlike top and bottom and front and back, left and right are not defined by the features of any structure. Nor are they properties of orientation in space that exist physically, independent of human perspective. They are spatial coordinates—paradoxically changing but ever unchanged—that always rely on a precise point of view for their meaning.

If we are standing side by side, for example, my right and left coincide with yours. No trouble there. If we face each other, on the other hand, they are exactly opposite: My right is on your left and vice versa. Both, however, still yield to instant calculation because our respective points of view are still accessible to each of us.

But if we attempt to reach agreement on the leftward or rightward location of something without orienting ourselves to a common reference point, trouble quickly sets in. We have only to remember the last time we tried to get directions to someone's house by phone to realize the truth of this. Our hostess told us to take a left turn at the corner market, but she meant *her* left, not ours, and so we ended up blocks away, out of patience and in a phone booth.

An exotic refinement of just this routine predicament forms the not-so-fanciful basis of what Martin Gardner calls *The Ozma Problem*. Gardner named it for the Ozma Project, one of the earliest attempts to communicate by radio telescope with other forms of life believed to exist somewhere in outer space. The interrelated problems of time and distance may be immense, but the question of what "language" to use, surprisingly enough, is a relatively simple matter. As Gardner points out, pictures of how life is lived on earth could simply be transmitted a dot at a time, much as newspaper wirephoto techniques do now. That is, you would use a binary code of radio pulses—ones and zeros, say, long and short—to connote filling in or leaving open spots on a grid like a sheet of grafting paper.

There is only one problem, the Ozma problem. We in the West would transmit the dots of our mosaic picture left to right. On receiving them, the alien world might align the dots right to left. No problem there, you say. Its inhabitants would simply have a *mirror image* of what we sent. Ah, but there *is* a problem there, the profoundest sort of problem, right there in that mirror image. What if their world were made of antimatter? Communicate we could, agrees Gardner with the relish of a man who loves a good thought twister, but visit each other we could not, under threat of instant obliteration.

How, then, are we to *know* if the other world is made of antimatter or not, if we mirror-image each other? *There is no way unless we can agree on left and right—and this we cannot do without a common point of reference.*

Can such a common reference point exist between us if we are in different solar systems, perhaps millions of light years apart?

It can and does exist, Gardner goes on to demonstrate, in the behavior of elementary particles as we have come to understand them since the fall of parity. But it wouldn't be fair to his book to reveal the solution to the Ozma problem here. Besides, the point we wish to make with this extended preamble is another one, a point central to the issue of how handedness in humans originates:

If it is hereditary as many scientists think, how can handedness—relying as it does on a precise orientation in space independent of any biological feature in the organism—be coded into the genes? Put another way, how does a gene know left from right?

No doubt the many potentialities of the human hand are inherited, as Abram Blau writes. The issue is whether their expression—throwing a ball, playing a violin, repairing a watch, painting, sculpting, manipulating a machine or scalpel—is destined from birth for one hand to the exclusion of the other.

Since the infant is not born with the full ability to exploit its innate manual capacity, that heritage strikes Blau as no more than "a promissory note maturing at some future date"[1] in a banking climate conducive to greater or lesser return. "The particular choice, direction, and nature of the skill finally achieved," as he puts it, "are quite outside the province of the germ plasm."[2]

But what about which hand is used? Is it, metaphorically

137

speaking, stipulated on the note or conditioned by the physical layout of the bank?

Blau leans to the latter. He cites studies of identical and fraternal twins in which, he contends, a far greater incidence of left-handedness should have occurred if the trait were genetic. After all, he emphasizes, both kinds of twin issue from a common gene pool, and identical twins from the same egg, or selection of genes. Yet the prevalence of sinistrality was only "slightly greater" than in the general population, plainly indicating "no definite correlation between biological symmetry and lateral preference."[3]

To find the answer to preferred handedness, he concludes, we must "enter the area of external environmental influences."[4]

Other researchers are not so sure. Nor have they been, in this century, ready to embrace such an all-or-nothing idea without reservation, although not all of them have been outspoken advocates of direct genetic transmission.

Early on, as we know, some of them favored eyedness as the indirect cause—until somebody thought to investigate handedness in those born blind and thereby forever destroyed that concept. Recent years, moreover, have seen a revival of interest in the old theory that speech originated in manual gestures and that cerebral lateralization evolved as a result. As Blau points out, function can determine structure just as structure can determine function.

Perhaps evolve it did, believers in a genetic base would grant. But nothing in that notion need be incompatible with the genes as a mechanism for that transmission. Genes, after all, are nature's vocabulary for just such an evolutionary statement.

Besides, hereditarians claim, twin data are conflicting. Other studies have shown a much higher incidence of left-handers in identical twins than in normal births. Furthermore, Hécaen and de Ajuriaguerra report from one relatively small study that sinistrality increases from 2 percent in children born to right-handers to 17 percent if the parents are mixed and to almost *half* if both are left-handed.

Such a progression, the two scientists agree, suggests a hereditary transmission of some sort.

But how are genetics to account for the birth of left-handers in completely right-handed families? And for that matter, how could handedness be related to which side of the brain language was on when it could be on *either* side in left-handers?

The simplest kind of genetic transmission—a single gene with left- and right-handed forms—was out of the question under these circumstances unless you assumed what the geneticist calls *partial penetrance,* weasel words meaning sometimes it has an effect and sometimes it doesn't.

Until recently these theoretical obstacles stood full in the path of what few genetic models were offered. Now, however, a couple of theories have come forward that skirt these roadblocks in a manner that tentatively satisfies hereditarians, if not environmentalists.

By far the "most ingenious and probably the most successful,"[5] in the words of even its critics, is the polygenetic (more than one gene) model by Jerre Levy and Thomas Nagylaki, a geneticist at the University of Wisconsin.

Levy and Nagylaki propose that handedness and brain lateralization are not only interrelated but jointly determined by two interacting genes instead of one, each having two possible forms of expression. One gene, they believe, determines which hemisphere will control language. The other gene determines whether the hand that hemisphere controls will be on the opposite side or the same side.

139

As might be expected, the idea of same-side control of the "language hand" has proved the most difficult aspect of their model for critics to swallow. Wasn't opposite-side control one of the mainstays of the vertebrate nervous systems?

It was the rule, but there were exceptions, Levy and Nagylaki decided—a deductive leap that cleared a hundred-year-old chasm and put the phenomenon of handedness squarely back in Broca's realm of brain organization again.

Was there any anatomical basis for such an assumption? There was, the two researchers argued. Existing postmortem data by Yakovlev and others on the "wiring" of the brain to the upper spinal cord revealed that in a few specimens less than half of the motor fibers crossed. Typically, eighty percent of the fibers do. Instead, in these exceptions most of the fibers ran straight down on the same side. What could more indicate same-side, rather than opposite-side, control?

"People who have language in the left side of the brain yet write with the left hand clearly must have access to those language centers in order to write," contends Levy. "There are only two ways they can do that. Either they're using same-side pathways or some form of relayed control across the commissures.

"Such a relayed control is simply unaesthetic to me—a stupid way to do it. I mean, if you've got language in the left hemisphere, why not just be right-handed? It doesn't make any biological sense."[6]

No, Levy's aesthetic sense told her, the reason they were left-handed with language in the left hemisphere was because a majority of their motor fibers failed to cross (decussate). Therefore, their same-side pathways, being biggest and hence dominant, made them as left-handed as those who had opposite-side control and language in their right hemispheres. Leaving aside to later the complication of brain damage, there were, in short, *two* distinct kinds of natural left-handers, those with same-side neural dominance and those with opposite-side.

Handedness, then, was not an isolated phenomenon. It was as intimately tied to the functional organization of the brain and nervous system as nature in her wisdom could make it.

Levy argues that the model works, that it accurately predicts "the number of left- and right-handed children born to parents who were both right-handed, both left-handed, or of opposite handedness."[7] Opponents of a genetic base concede this fit is acceptable—if Levy and Nagylaki are allowed their own "suitable"[8] pick of parameters. But they dispute the model on grounds that it cannot account for the unexpectedly low number of left-handers among siblings and twins, particularly those that are identical.

They brush aside the hereditarian claim that special mirror-image effects and frequent prenatal pathology among twins distort their statistical contribution. Nonsense, they charge, twins from a single egg should *always* have the same handedness since they have the very same genes— *if* the cause is genetic.

Instead, they point out, what do we find? That the number of discordant cases is so high that it suggests "that handedness within generations is very largely a matter of chance."[9]

If a genetic influence exists, they conclude, it is certainly "dwarfed by a large random component"[10]—a fact at least recognized by the other genetic model currently in vogue, that of England's Marian Annett, a Hull University psychologist.

Annett's model touches just about all theoretical bases. It holds that humans are not "left-handed" or "right-handed," really, any more than they are simply "short" or "tall." Rather, she likes to think, they demonstrate a variety of hand skills that is generally continuous across the broadest possible range, from fully right to fully left.

Although this sounds suspiciously like the traits of height and weight—which are determined by not just one gene but many—Annett insists it is due to "accidental"[11] influences on early development both before and after birth, for example in the handling of the child. The same is true, in a more restricted sense, of all asymmetric vertebrates. For complex statistical reasons, that factor can be expected to produce the essentially random split in paw preference among lesser animals when narrowed to a single task for testing.

In humans, however, says Annett, this distribution as a whole is displaced by a pronounced "shift" to the right because of a second factor, one "possibly genetic but modified by cultural influences."[12] That factor, she believes, may be something as simple as a single gene which, if you have it, dictates the rightward shift, but whose absence throws you back onto the random forces that determine your place in the normal distribution.

Thus the natural cause of left-handedness would be founded upon, as two other environmentally minded researchers put it, "an inherited absence of the predisposition to be right-handed."[13]

But again, how is such a predisposition to be coded into a microscopic bit of germ plasm?

Under the best of circumstances, it seems, people have trouble telling left from right. Barely a quarter of five-year-old English school children tested in one experiment could distinguish between their two hands in use. This might be dismissed as a question of maturity were it limited to the early years. But the difficulty appears not only ageless but spread across cultures and curiously selective in its victims.

Women, for example, do significantly worse than men on identifying pictures of body parts as belonging to one side or the other. Researchers have suggested this is because they tend to be deficient in the visual-spatial functions of the right hemisphere.

This distinction seems indirectly borne out in the visual match of words to pictures by men. They do better on those requiring a verbal response of "right," a throwback, one research team speculates, to the fact that they probably first learn which is their right by the hand they are taught to "write" with. (The subjects were all right-handed.) But the difference disappears completely when visual arrows are substituted for words, (right-hemisphere) image for (left-hemisphere) symbol.

On the other hand, what are we to make of the fact that native Arabs and Hebrews make *five times* as many errors as Israeli immigrants in following oral commands that require a right or left orientation, one of them as deceptively simple as "Look to the left" or "Look to the right"?

Researcher Martin Albert decided the answer lay in the reverse right-to-left direction of written Arabic and Hebrew. Western left-to-right reading activates *both* brain hemispheres, Albert knew, the left for understanding language, the right for motor control of the eye movement. Since the eyes move in the opposite direction in Semitic reading, Albert realized the left hemisphere must do both jobs. As a consequence, he decided, the spatially specialized right hemisphere was left totally out of it and never got the incessant practice in right-left orientation that Western reading affords.

Varied though such factors be—age, sex, culture—they

143

illustrate the sensitivity of our left-right orientation. And by implication, they suggest to some environmentalists a nongenetic nature in our choice of hand.

Michael Corballis and Ivan Beale of McGill University in Montreal, unlike Yakovlev, contend that the human nervous system is not biased to one side or the other by the crossing, or failure to cross, of its neural fibers. Like all vertebrates, they believe, man has "approximate bilateral symmetry,"[14] enough at any rate to account for his inability to discern natural reality from its mirror image. Why else, they ask, would he at his most intelligent shrink fearfully back from the hand of friendship if it belonged to some seemingly humanlike (but careful: antimatter!) traveler from outer space?

He shrinks back, Corballis and Beale insist, because he cannot tell the difference. And he cannot tell the difference because, deep down inside his brain where it really counts, he has no inherent way to tell the difference.

Although the exact mechanism and form of our memory remain a mystery, these researchers further suggest it may even be that *every* memory trace laid down for a given stimulus *simultaneously and automatically engraves a (ghostly?) mirror image* on the opposite side of the brain, using the commissures as its means of transmission.

"Such connections would create a kind of neural mirror that serves to 'reflect' . . . across the midline," Corballis and Beale write. "If a trace is established in one hemisphere, its mirror image will be established in the other."[15]

As they point out, a wealth of inferential evidence from experimental animals supports this view. To name just one instance, Pavlov, the father of conditioning, could teach a dog *not* to salivate when touched on one side of its body. Once that was done, however, Pavlov could not teach the

144

same dog to salivate when it was touched at the same (mirror-image) point on the other side. Why? The answer lies in the inherent confusion between mirror-image memory traces etched in the two hemispheres, Corballis and Beale argue. How do they know? Because Pavlov found he could eliminate that confusion in his salivating dog by *cutting the corpus callosum*—in effect, blocking the duplication.

It could equally be argued, of course, that by cutting the callosum, Pavlov created two separate brains, each of which could be taught a different response without interference from the other. But John Noble of the University of London first taught a mirror-image discrimination task to one hemisphere of a monkey, then severed its callosum. Tested on which image it preferred with its untrained hemisphere, the monkey immediately showed a preference not for the original stimulus but *for its mirror image,* indicating that a reverse impression most likely had been laid down.

Monkeys and dogs are one thing, hereditarians would point out, humans quite another. What reason do we have to believe that we also duplicate memory traces in mirror-image form?

Asked to describe pictures of various faces viewed thirty minutes before, the two researchers counter, subjects in one experiment were wrong *over a third of the time* on which profile they saw. Other investigators have found people just as likely to recognize a mirror image as the original—and often unable to remember which they saw when both are presented after the trial to refresh their memory. Corballis and Beale believe that such confusion is "at least consistent with the interpretation that memory traces tend to be duplicated in mirror-image form."[16]

Such a neural mix-up may even be reflected in the curious phenomenon of *mirror writing,* that upside-down-inside-out script of which Leonardo da Vinci was our most illustrious practitioner. Indeed, another Canadian researcher has found that right-handers asked to switch to their left usually do better at mirror-writing than normal writing—indicating their trained hemisphere is still trying to run things, albeit at cross purposes and with Alice in Wonderland results.

Paradoxically, Austrian physicist Ernst Mach speculated in the last century that mirror image problems in symmetry might be solved not by sensory or perceptual means but by *motor* acts such as writing. Corballis and Beale doubt that the laws of motion, Wigner and the fall of parity notwithstanding, contribute all that much to the asymmetry of handedness. But Jerome Bruner sees a suggestive link between the manipulation of language and the tool use that Yakovlev mounts so much of his arresting theory upon.

The right hemisphere of our brain holds the context of thought while the left works on it to produce speech, says Bruner, just as one hand usually holds the material being worked and the other hand the tool. The possible relationship between opposite hemispheres and opposite hands is tantalizing since man through his tools and language is responsible for so much of the world's visible violation of theoretic (mirror) symmetry.

Nevertheless, according to Corballis and Michael Morgan of Cambridge, the alleged influence of the asymmetric brain upon hand preference as a strict consequence of genetic predetermination is illusory. Their interpretation of the possible relationship between two brains and two hands is "rather more prosaic"[17] than the hereditarians'.

In their view, the fact that the right hemisphere generally lacks both expressive language and control of the dominant hand means not that it is specialized for other things—

"normal, even elementary, perceptual processes"[18]—but that it is simply retarded developmentally. That relative retardation, they feel, is a consequence of a "fairly general left to right" organic and functional maturation that "normally favors earlier or more rapid development on the left than on the right."[19]

That principle, they contend, is typical of biological asymmetries in the animal world as varied as the left-side-specific nerve control of birdsong in the chaffinch, the surviving left ovaries and oviducts of most other birds, and the single left tusk of the narwhal. A predominant left-right gradient in strength and hardiness is reflected, too, in how the right side of a structural symmetry seems almost "programmed" sometimes to wither away internally while the left robustly survives. If a hair is tied around the middle of a newt's embryo, for example, "Siamese twins" are produced in which the left is usually normal, the right is not.

Such asymmetries are essentially developmental, Corballis and Morgan declare. They are thought to be coded, not in the chromosomes, but in the protoplasm outside the nucleus of the egg (cytoplasm). Genes may express or modify the results of the maturational cycles they embody, but genes do not determine their direction.

Hence, say Corballis and Morgan, both language and handedness may issue out of the left hemisphere's dominance—but as byproducts of its more rapid development, not as an unfolding of genetic promise.

Jerre Levy, for one, vigorously disagrees. "What they don't seem to understand is that what is in the cytoplasm of the egg cell are *gene products of the mother,* just one generation delay in genetic control. It makes no difference which. It's still genetic."[20]

Almost lost in the intricacies of the argument are two of

Corballis and Morgan's corollary conclusions. For one thing, they concede that some people, perhaps because of a recessive gene, may lack any consistent cerebral asymmetry. Their handedness may be determined at random, perhaps by Annett's hypothesized shift. For another thing, their idea as to where this comes from smacks strongly of Yakovlev and Wigner.

It conceivably could be, they suggest, "a universal biological phenomenon" based on "the asymmetry in the molecular structure of living tissue."[21]

What about left-handedness as a possible consequence of injury, what psychologists call, with a fine sense of nuance, brain "insult"?

Since left-handers relentlessly continue to be born to right-handed parents, Canadian psychologist Paul Bakan has decided the phenomenon must be a side effect of stressful birth. True, most left handers are perfectly normal physically and mentally, Bakan emphasizes (a point the less scientific majority may wish to dispute). But he finds a significantly higher percentage of them among those most often adversely affected by difficult delivery: males in general, and children born to women over thirty, who are past their child-bearing prime and far more susceptible to defective offspring.

The culprit, Bakan is convinced, is that same reduced flow of oxygen during the crucial process of birth that many researchers now think leads to stammering and later difficulties in reading and writing. Despite his artful demurrer, which makes of their anomaly a harmless neurological "guilt by association," Bakan is talking about brain damage. He hypothesizes (since it is too subtle ever to be found) a slight injury to the left hemisphere.

Subtly traumatized at birth, he believes, the left hemisphere, while openly manifesting its hurt through any one or more eventual deficits in expressive language, secretly forfeits its manual dominance to the right hemisphere and thereby the left hand. Though various forms of training and conditioning in a right-handed society will inevitably mitigate what follows, the result is virtually immutable: someone who is more or less left-handed.

Most researchers, however, believe Bakan's theory is grossly exaggerated. As neuropsychologist Paul Satz of Florida University puts it, "If a phenomenon such as pathological left-handedness exists, then what about the converse effect—namely pathological right-handedness?

" . . . if brain lesions are random in nature, then there must be cases of right hemisphere damage in natural left-handers who [therefore] are predisposed to become manifest right-handers"[22] of inferior spatial abilities.

Alas, we are still looking for *them*.

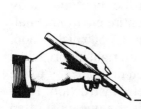

Who's Left-Handed, Anyway?

13

In *The New England Journal of Medicine,* a doctor from Missouri attempted to settle once and for all the question of how to tell if you're a left-hander. It was easy, he said. You just hold your thumbs up side by side and look at the base of the nails. The one on the dominant hand is usually wider and squarer.

Would that it were that simple. But alas, as we have seen, even that little bit of dominance can be all but qualified out of existence. There really *is* no easy answer. For as Abram Blau writes, the issue is now and forever confused by the same lingering question: left-handed in *what?*

Estimates of left-handedness, in fact, range from almost fifty percent down to one percent, depending on the criteria used. Of 250 students whose handedness was clinically tested by one researcher, only 19 were right-handed in all the tasks he bothered to check. If his criteria for establishing handedness were adopted by that majority of researchers who insist that right-handedness is an all-or-nothing proposition, the net result would be an almost exact reversal of the generally accepted handedness profile of our society today: Only about 7½ percent of the population would be classified as right-handers!

The issue, as Blau points out, is further confounded by the age-old factors that underpin the entire environmentalist position—socialization and training. Of 500 high school boys Blau tested, the ratio of left to right approached chance in simple tasks, but was skewed dramatically to the right on those requiring long and careful instruction. Paramount among such tasks, of course, is the one most often used in attempting to determine handedness: handwriting, ironically the most "overlearned" complex manual act in man's vast armamentarium of acquired skills.

Is the prevailing rightward bias of handwriting due to the fact that it demands the most of our head and hand—and nervous system—and thus draws most heavily on our natural propensity for putting our best side forward?

Or is it because the skill is relentlessly taught and therefore highly vulnerable to the kind of pedantry that too easily slips over the line into outright indoctrination?

Blau, on the issue an environmentalist at heart, concludes, "The individual is influenced more by the right-handedness of the world he lives in than by any hypothetical, intrinisic element."[1] With obvious relish he reports one study in which sixteen of thirty-four second-graders in one school were found to write left-handed. Why such a phenomenal proportion? It was simple, said Blau, and far-reaching in its implications. Both their first- and second-grade teachers, as it happened, wrote with their left hands too!

Lately I have been looking at some of my left-handed

friends—and wondering just what psychology would make of them. If you gathered them up for a picnic on the beach at Point Reyes—an outing we planned but never quite consummated—you would detect in their overall demeanor nothing very exceptional one way or another except, perhaps, how they threw a Frisbee or drew their beer and lemonade.

Even then, I'm betting, their anomalous nature would for most of the day escape your notice, so varied and widespread is its manual expression.

The group is composed of seven males and three females, ranging in age from their early forties down to a schoolboy in his early teens. Vocationally they include a food company executive, a musician-carpenter, an actor-director, a jewelrymaker, a nurse, a homemaker-seamstress, a psychologist, and the administrator of a small federal agency. Taking us together, all but I remain resolutely left-handed in writing. But then none of them went to elementary school in the 1930s, when the scholastic war on sinistrals reached its fever pitch.

Their united front is deceptive, however. Behind it, their diverse manual preferences fall into the same mixed bag psychology has come to expect. On some twenty tasks I bothered to ask about, none of them proved entirely left-handed, and not one of them was exactly like the other.

Their left-handed responses ranged from a high of all nine on tennis (though one spoiled my questionnaire's symmetry by perversely playing Ping-Pong with her right) to a low of four on batting a baseball. Left-handers are usually not discouraged from hitting on that side, of course. As any sandlotter knows, it gives you a half step head start in running to first base. Indeed, right-handers are often switched by coaches for that reason.

Why so many of my left-handed friends reacted just the

opposite like I did is something I don't know, unless it was somehow neurologically ordained. (Three are right-eyed, two mixed, so this doesn't seem a factor.) Perhaps it's just another example of the stubbornness that led Blau to label them mavericks.

Similarly, using scissors or drawing a cork is done left-handed by only half of them, probably because each implement is engineered to favor right-handers and can be at least adequately learned by switching left-handers, in spite of their innate (if it is innate) preference.

Curiously though, only half of my friends said they unscrewed lids with their left hand, a task that often requires the greater manual strength normally residing in the hand you prefer. Three of the others said they used either hand, while two reported they preferred their right.

In only two kinds of tasks did none of them prefer the right hand: hammering, and using a razor (the men) or lipstick (the women). In each of these tasks there was one person who said he (or she) *had* no preference.

Indeed, "either" was a more common response across the full range of tasks than "right," although all but one performed at least one task with the right hand. Most of them were right-handed in three or four, and one in as many as five. I was the only left-hander who betrayed not a jot of ambidextrality.

Anomalies to begin with, in small ways my sinister friends *stayed* anomalies within their renegade band itself. In addition to the woman whose handedness was strangely divided in Ping-Pong and tennis, one man threw overhand with his left hand but underhand with his right.

Eyedness and footedness were no statistical help, either. Six of us kicked with our left foot, two with our right, and two with either. Only one among us was left-eyed—a far rarer preference normally, anyway, for some reason—but

154

two said they used either eye in sighting through a telescope, gunsight, or keyhole.

If such an informal sampling seems hopelessly muddled, formal studies by professionals trained in steering through the treacherous shoals of statistics are no more clear-cut— for *either* hand.

According to Hécaen and de Ajuriaguerra, who surveyed all the major research, people themselves often don't know what to tell researchers. In one survey on the supposedly straight-forward matter of which hand they were better with, the subjects were wrong in *a quarter to half the cases* where the truth of their assertion was experimentally tested. A simple question like "Are you left-handed?" generally elicits answers that neglect such incidental but untaught tasks as which hand you use in brushing your teeth or striking a match.

If people don't know what to make of the questions, how can psychologists know what to make of their answers? Part of the problem arises out of definition. One psychologist defines handedness in terms of the hand preferred in learning new tasks. Another defines it in terms of the one that excels in fine and precise movements, such as threading a needle. Still others define it in terms of relative strength and dexterity of the two hands.

Almost none of them can agree on how to phrase a questionnaire so as to winnow out crucial distinctions. How, for example, do you distinguish between ambidextrous and ambilateral? Ambidextrous applies to those who have not yet established a dominant hand but can use both with the same facility most people have in their preferred hand. Ambilateral, on the other hand, is generally applied to those who have not established a dominant hand and cannot use *either* well.

Obviously, such distinctions must always be used with

155

care. But both can be loosely covered by the simple response "either." How are such important differences to be gotten across to people filling out a questionnaire?

For that matter, the use of *any* questionnaire can be faulted seriously on several other fronts, chief among them the items selected and their comparative worth. Take, for example, eating habits. "The British . . . have the odd habit of using their knife and fork at meal times simultaneously . . . holding the knife in the right, and the fork in the left . . ." says one researcher.

"Cricket bats are not commonly used in Parisian suburbs, and many inhabitants of Manhattan apartment blocks find little use for rakes. While most men make shift to sew on indispensable buttons, the use of needle and thread is unquestionably far more prevalent among the female sex."[2] In short, if the needle is included, what about the hammer?

That same writer confessed himself nonplussed to find that one perfectly fine-appearing item for possible handedness testing—wielding a broom and rake—was in reality a veritable witches' fen of psychic confabulation. "It would seem that holding these tools with the left hand at the top, and thereby sweeping or raking a region to the right of the operator is fairly widespread," he reported. "This could, perhaps, be attributed to a general tendency to favor the right half of space as far as perception and attention go.

"But . . . I have found . . . many people use brooms and rakes either way round, changing hands accordingly."[3]

Dealing cards, he added, could likewise be misleading because a surprising number of right-handers hold the pack in their *right* hand and deal with their left: "One thoroughly right-handed man told me that he had acquired the habit of dealing left-handed by simply copying his father, who had first taught him card games."[4]

156

In fact, one pair of researchers argues, the more direct the investigation, the more numerous the tests, and the less they concern learned movements, the larger the proportion of left-handedness.

But again, a lot depends on how the researcher and his subjects cooperate to define left-handedness—or more exactly, on how they choose to distinguish between left-handedness and mixed, or undecided, handedness.

One does not find an increase in the number of left-handed subjects, Hécaen and de Ajuriaguerra contend in the fact of contradictory evidence, but rather an increase in the number of subjects whose right- and left-sidedness is confused.

Such frustrations have only multiplied, not lessened, the number of incidental tasks seized upon by inventive researchers as possible unconscious indicators of true handedness, assuming that exists. Investigators have kept a weather eye on such diverse chores as carrying luggage, purses, and umbrellas, both rolled and unrolled.

One of the most intriguing and potentially helpful new tests, if it proves out, has been developed by Theodore H. Blau. Called the Torque Test, it has a child draw some X's, circle them, and sign his name, first with one hand, then the other. The strength and control in handwriting indicates the preferred hand, Blau reports, but the drawing of the circles indicates something else: the brain organization underlying the child's natural tendency before the onset of socialization. In other words, the child may do many or most things with his right hand, yet be a left-hander at heart. How does Blau determine this? Simple, he says. Right-handers consistently draw their circles counterclockwise, left-handers tend to draw them clockwise.

But even if researchers could agree once and for all upon a set of abilities as most truly indicative of handedness (whatever *that* is), bypassing preference-by-questionnaire in favor of behavior-by-test would not in itself instantly dissolve all difficulties. In some measures—the manual speed involved in moving pegs, for example—practice improves the performance of both hands without eliminating the difference between them. True enough. Retesting on motor tasks, however, yields a positive, dependable relationship between the two hands *less than a third of the time,* indicating that these measures are nowhere near as reliable as the canons of responsible research ordinarily require.

When the movements are not simply graded muscular contractions made either for speed or accuracy but complexly programmed and timed sequences—such as, for example, knitting—training is a distorting factor unless it has been given to *both* hands without a scintilla of favoritism. Any hint that one hand has been given more practice than the other and all data can be thrown out the window.

The *kind* of task is critical, too. In one study, depending on which of three measures were used to make the identification, the percentage of left-handers ranged from *two to thirty-five percent.*

Then, too, a motor task as simple as flexing a single finger can throw the statistician into a quandry. Right-handers are better at it—*but with their left hand,* which led one researcher to decide that the control of fine movement had nothing to do with hand preference!

No wonder one neurophysiologist, attempting to amass a hundred cases from seven different sources of handedness data to study language loss by hemisphere, felt impelled to point out that some of what he found could not be accepted as "valid indications of sinistrality."[5]

Worst of all, not only does performance frequently disagree with expressed preference, what people *say* about which hand they use on a given task *one time* may not agree with what they say the next. One research team found that fully a *fifth* of those they questioned had changed their minds, either consciously or unconsciously, on a significant number of items when questioned again. Self-styled left-handers, wouldn't you know it, were the most frequent offenders.

Under such circumstances, it is somewhat less than enlightening to learn that results of both questionnaire and test alike not only conflict, but can vary with age, sex, and geography—not to mention with who is doing the testing.

Left-handed classification seldom changes in the adult years, says one researcher, nor do the proportions in childhood. But another claims he found almost twice as many in a group of four- to fourteen-year-olds than in a group of eight- to fourteen-year-olds. To add to experimenter frustration, some tests yield an increase in dextrality with age, others an increase in sinistrality, prompting the observer to something like the sentiment expressed by President Kennedy when two emissaries—one civilian, one military—returned from separate fact-finding trips to Vietnam with diametrically opposing reports on the war:

"Are you gentlemen sure you didn't go to different countries?"[6]

Pity the poor researcher, then, who found, in testing one group of normal students, that *twenty percent were left-handed,* while in another comparable group he found exactly *none.* Seeking to straighten out his perspective, he then compared two classes of the learning disabled. There he discovered sixty-six percent and *1.2 percent*—and neither class was in any way set up differently from the other.

At that, it can be worse. In a test of fifty-seven children between the ages of five and a half and thirteen, another researcher found a left-hand superiority in sixteen of them. A year later he went back—and found it in only one.

Artists, Oddballs, or Inferiors?

14

Left-handers—writes one of them, James De Kay—have a "maddening habit of thinking in elipses rather than straight lines. Their train of thought is apt to meander through the whole alphabet on the way from A to B." Not only is left-handed thinking inelegant, tortuous, and without grace, he observes, its essential illogic profusely produces such odd associations as "did you know that a Camel cigarette is exactly the same length as the width of Todd-AO movie film?"[1]

At the same time, De Kay adds, left-handers "spell like half-drunk Elizabethan typesetters" and betray an all but unmistakable offbeat demeanor in which "a certain frowziness may be involved—a vagrant cowlick, a missing button, an unfocused gaze, inarticulateness, a tendency to mumble . . ."[2]

Such humorous if overstated generalizations, need it be

said, don't always apply to every left-hander. But each contains a kernel of important truth. The artistic, the oddball, the slow or disabled in learning—all include a higher proportion of left-handers than chance alone would dictate. Why?

We know more about their susceptibility to learning problems than we do about their penchant for eccentric or creative behavior, of course. The need for successful schooling has until recently made such knowledge the more imperative. But now we know our head is wired to give us, literally, two different brains that function independently and do different kinds of tasks. Thanks to the split-brain experiments, we are aware, too, that each is intimately tied to a specific hand.

As a result, even passing inferences as casual as De Kay's begin to suggest the deepest sort of relationship between hand use and the cognitive character of the controlling hemisphere, between the hand we tend to act with and the "brain" we tend to think with.

For that reason, it might be argued, left-handers are more likely than right-handers to be on intimate terms with the visual, spatial, and imagistic gifts of the right hemisphere; with the raw material of art itself; with perception. Conversely, it would seem to follow, they would be less likely than right-handers to be all that strongly in touch with the expressive gift of abstraction and the raw materials of science, language, and math.

Standing all but speechless in a world of symbols, their attention turned silently inward on the teeming images of sight, sound, and touch that flit across their minds—goes the argument—why *wouldn't* they appear maverick in the eyes of a conventional, "with-it" (right-handed) society?

As persuasive as such thoughts may at first blush be, the issue is not that simple. It is certainly, however, worth our

closest examination. Let us begin with what we suspect—
and go on from there to what we know.

For openers, De Kay's whimsical description of typical
left-handed thinking sounds very much like the right hemisphere dominantly in action. By its very nature, it relies on
the perceptual images of touch, sound, and sight, not on
language. Being essentially perceptual rather than abstract,
it cannot help but kick over the traces of linearity when it
fuses these images into simultaneous patterns—neural *ge-
stalts,* mental pictures of reality.

Unlike letters, these pictures need not be sequential in
their intrinsic components to achieve meaning. Each is holistic, all of a piece. The act of putting any two of them
together obeys no known law of logic. It can be purely comparative, relational, juxtaposed in terms of the thinker's
unique life experience.

No wonder then that such a process—unspoken as it often is until after the fact—often strikes the right-hander as
illogical!

If such activity further strikes the right-hander as unworthy of his grand notions of intelligence, he would do
well to read the remarks of respected physicists like Murray Gell-Mann. Gell-Mann stresses the importance of per-
ceiving *apparent patterns* in natural phenomena before
attempting to theorize, conceptualize, about what such
phenomena *mean.* In other words, he counsels us to give
priority to our right hemispheres.

When we do—not "pushing the river," but waiting for it
to cast up its secret treasure on the shores of our awareness—the result is often the kind of fruitful connection between seemingly unrelated bits of information that charac-
terizes inventive or creative thought.

Many, if not all, commercially marketed techniques of

"brainstorming" that have grown out of the "think tank" approach to problem solving are built around exactly this premise: that answers take definite form out of the amorphous swirl of right-hemisphere sensory impressions.

Educator William J. J. Gordon, for example, calls his system *Synectics,* from the Greek word for joining together different and apparently irrelevant elements. Synectics asks that we stay perceptually alive to all facets of a problem by looking for the strange in the ordinary and the ordinary in the strange. It cautions us to refrain from foreclosing too quickly on seemingly farfetched answers that well up pell-mell but unbidden and strike us as illogical or too easy. It advises us above all to "think metaphorically," to *visualize* in our minds, to *picture* solutions in concrete terms rather than endlessly talking about alternatives.

All these steps, obviously, are grounded in the speechless imagistic processes of the right hemisphere—and haven't we learned that it controls the left hand? As Jerome Bruner poetically suggests, doesn't the left hand *know more creatively* than the right?

Writes James De Kay about those two preeminent left-handers, Ben Franklin and the man Michael Barsley refers to as "the patron saint of the sinistrals,"[3] Leonardo da Vinci:

> Leonardo's friends all knew man would never fly, yet by putting ideas together in his own way he designed a rig that apparently *could* have flown. As for Ben's rocking chair, if it wasn't a left-handed conception, why hadn't it occurred to anyone before to combine those ancient artifacts, the chair and the cradle?[4]

People as diverse in discipline and interest as art teacher Ann O'Hanlon of Mill Valley, California, and famed attorney Louis Nizer have put the left hand powerfully to work in ways that prove the truth of Bruner's observations about art—and Jung's about the "unconscious."

Nizer, a right-hander, has long had the habit of casually, aimlessly, all-but-unconsciously sketching jurers with his left hand while listening to testimony. Such sketches, he finds, give him surprising—and useful—insights into the personality and character of those upon whom his client's fate depends. So effective have such intuitions proven in tailoring his presentation and summary that Nizer keeps a file of the sketches.

O'Hanlon, dismayed at the rigid ineffectual performance by a summer art class of nuns years ago, on impulse instructed them to switch to their left hands. (Unknown to her, the technique has an honorable Renaissance history. Masters then had their pupils change hands to seduce from them a freer, more imaginative line.)

The result was better art—and, says O'Hanlon, more relaxed, creative people. She still encourages her pupils to use the left hand, sometimes both hands at once—and gets in return convincing visual evidence of what neuroscientists now know: that each hemisphere of the brain not only "sees" different things, it "sees" things differently.

But hold on. The careful reader will realize we are talking about two different things here. Nizer is right-handed; so are the students O'Hanlon asks to switch. She has never, in her memory, asked a left-hander to change to the right hand. So we are talking not about left-handers but about right-handers. We are referring, in fact, to the *left hands of right-handers,* people who write with their right hands, not with their left.

If we know anything, we know that the left hand of the right-hander is controlled by the non-linguistic, or spatial, hemisphere. Can the same be said for the left hand of the left-hander?

Not exactly. Since that hand does the writing, it must have access to language—and by all the canons of brain research, that access cannot help but interfere with spatial abilities.

Indeed, we know that left-handers are not uniformly lacking in language. Some have used words with a vengeance. As De Kay notes about Lewis Carroll's most famous story:

> *Through the Looking glass* is the most left-handed book ever written. The world behind the mirror is opposite in every way from Alice's (right-handed) real world—corkscrews turn the wrong way, queens stand on the wrong side of kings—and of course there is "Jabberwocky," Carroll's great masterpiece of word play.[5]

(Although De Kay fails to mention it, the fact that Carroll was a professor of mathematics at Oxford assumes perhaps added significance in view of parity and the subtle handedness of molecules.)

How can it be, then, in the words of University of Minnesota researcher Bryng Bryngelson, who has studied left-handers for over thirty-five years, that as a group they are more "highly imaginative, creative and socially sensitive"[6] than right-handers?

We don't know, really. Another school of thought would probably say that Bryngelson offers a clue in his contrasting remarks about right-handers. He found them "more outgoing and extroverted,"[7] which is just another way of saying left-handers are more private and introverted—in a society

166

that prides itelf on the Rotarian virtues of glad-handing, definitely oddball.

Indeed, studies have shown that left-handers are more "oppositional" or contrary in their natures. Coerced as they are from childhood on by a conformist world of insistent right-handers, why shouldn't they be? "A child who overcomes the pressures of society . . . and persists in left-handedness," writes Blau, may "develop a streak of stubbornness or an inclination to go against group pressure and accepted norms."[8]

Whatever its source, he adds, that negativity can breed "a willingness to go it alone in spite of other people's objections—as we have seen in Presidents Ford and Truman.

"Who would have thought that easy-going Truman would have dropped the bomb or that President Ford would have pardoned Mr. Nixon so soon?"[9]

Are left-handers as a group neurologically inferior?

The White House may have thought so. President Ford bumped his head and tumbled down airplane ramps so many times that his staff reportedly put an election-year embargo on official press pictures and handouts of such embarrassing events. Then again, perhaps they were motivated by fear of the sentiment expressed by the former quarterback on Mr. Ford's high school football team, a professor of psychology named Allan Elliott. Although Ford purportedly only *writes* left-handed, the president, said Elliott, was "pretty left-handed" in his high school days and "we used to say jokingly that he even thought left-handed."[10]

At that, although left-handers often exhibit high degrees of motor control and finesse (as anyone knows who has

167

ever watched Jimmy Connors play tennis), the notion persists that left-handers are somehow neurologically out of register, undependable, unstable. In baseball, for example, southpaw pitchers are traditionally feared as dangerously, killingly wild.

Those who traffic in the myth of left-handed erraticism in sports turn a deaf ear also to the offbeat abilities of Pete Gray, when and if they ever hear of him. Called The One-Armed Wonder, Pete Gray played five years of professional baseball, one with the World Champion Saint Louis Browns, during the Second World War. Since childhood, Gray had hit, caught, and thrown with his left arm. He swung a heavy thirty-eight-ounce bat with authority and frequently threw out base runners who dared take liberties with his handicap. As sportswriter Jack Cavanaugh describes it:

> After catching a fly ball, Gray, using one swift, fluid motion, would bring his glove up to his right armpit, letting the ball roll down his wrist and across his chest. With his glove tucked under his right stump, he would then drop his left hand in time to catch the ball and then rifle it in.[11]

Not all left-handers are retarded or brain-damaged in the clinical sense, of course, and not all retarded or brain-damaged are left-handed. But it is a doleful fact that left-handedness does pop up more frequently among the ranks of the defective. Undoubtedly the mixed criteria for handedness used in making such classifications render any hard figure suspect. And for that matter, how could the percentages be otherwise loaded? Left-handers are bound to dominate these statistics, some researchers contend, if only because birth accidents are in no way selective in what

168

hemisphere they strike. Any injury-forced switch in function from one side of the brain to the other will, as a matter of course, reflect the disproportionate number of right-handers turned into left-handers, assuming for the sake of argument that neuroscientists are correct when they agree that more people are naturally right- than left-handed.

As a result of arithmetic alone, therefore, left-handers are doomed to suffer what one researcher perceptively calls "a bad press."[12]

Nevertheless, suspicion lingers in some scientific and educational quarters that such a bad press is at least partly justified. For left-handedness has been statistically, clinically, and experimentally linked with just about every kind of human ailment, foible, and deficiency from bed-wetting to alexia (word blindness).

Paul Bakan, for example, reports an incidence of left-handedness among a group of male alcoholics almost *twice* what might have been expected from matching their composite profile against the national average. To him, naturally, given his theoretic bias, the figure suggests that fetal oxygen starvation may prove "a precursor of alcoholism."[13]

But if such pathology does exist at birth, other research indirectly indicates, it may be less a matter of outright tissue damage than what might be called a functionally-induced neural "short circuit," or to be more accurate, what is called a "phase distortion" in electronics—a situation in which each channel of a stereo, for example, plays fine on its own but discordantly together.

In such instances, neurologically speaking, the two cerebral hemispheres may be equally "out of sync." Neither side may be clearly in control of its specialty. Both may compete across the commissures for dominance. The result: a subsequent loss in cerebral efficiency and effectiveness, a growing neural friction and trauma.

Researchers here and abroad, interestingly enough, have hinted as much about schizophrenia. Noting a preponderance of hospitalized child and adult schizophrenics with mixed or conflicting lateral preferences in hand-eye usage but no signs of anatomical damage or mental deterioration, they concluded that such mixed preferences must be due to a primary "dysfunction" of the central nervous system.

In other words, there was nothing materially wrong with the schizophrenic's cerebral equipment. It was somehow out of phase, just not working properly.

As it happens, left-handers figured less prominently in such research than mixed right-handers/left-eyers. Then, too, neither study in any way proved that schizophrenia was the *effect* of such an imbalance. It may very well have been the cause. But the notion of some sort of neural mix-up, a conflictive dominance, impeding performance in an otherwise normal-seeming brain has enormous investigative appeal in the light of such diverse problems as bed-wetting, alexia, and stammering.

Indeed, according to a theory by Abram Blau, left-handers often wet their beds well past the first formative years because *both* hemispheres of their brain send messages to the bladder to open and close. The poor confused bladder, Blau thinks, not knowing which hemisphere is in charge, freezes at the critical instant.

As for alexia and stammering, a similar "war" between the hemispheres has been well established. Alexics read *d* for *b* and *p* for *q* and confuse words like "was" and "saw." They do this, evidently, because the wrong hemisphere suddenly seizes directional control of the linear process. As might be expected, EEG readings show the hemispheres of alexic children to be far less synchronized electrically than normal. The two sides of their brain, in short, are out of phase.

In much the same manner, if not crisply lateralized in its function, either hemisphere can wrestle with the other over which will "do the talking." The stammer resulting from this neural tug-of-war reveals more clearly than words that in some people *both* hemispheres take command—at one and the same time. Once understood, such an anomaly makes clear how a mother could lament that her son couldn't play ball because "[being] left-handed [he was] never certain from which direction a ball was coming."[14]

Since the left-hander is more often implicated in all these admittedly minor offenses against normality than the right-hander, it appears our long-standing suspicions are in part confirmed: His brain is not always as cleanly separated into two independent hemispheres, each of which in its function ordinarily respects the autonomy and expertise of the other.

On the contrary, the hemispheres of such weakly lateralized left-handers appear to fight like cats and dogs for cerebral dominance. Not only do they battle over which will do what, they also are believed to invade each other's neural turf—language especially—to spread their specialty.

Such an attempt invariably interferes with the other hemisphere's exercise of its particular talents—as Levy found when she tested and compared the verbal and spatial skills of matched groups of left- and right-handed males at the California Institute of Technology.

The verbal and spatial IQs of the right-handers were 138 and 130, respectively—an inconsiderable difference between the relative performances of the two hemispheres. But those of the left-handers were 142 and 117—a discrepancy *three times* as great.

Clearly, Levy concluded, the left-handers were not only

verbally superior (a surprising result in view of our earlier speculation about the hemisphere-hand relationship), but owed much of that superiority to augmentation from the other hemisphere. Judging by the test results, the other hemisphere had been "recruited" to language processing at the cost of depressing its natural spatial abilities.

Years later another researcher conducted a similar experiment with kindergarten children—and demonstrated that no significant differences existed between the two kinds of IQ for five- and six-year-olds of either sex or handedness. Did this mean that in left-handers the invasion of the spatial hemisphere by language occurs only in response to the progressive and growing demands of an education system overwhelmingly grounded in the manipulation of symbols?

Did it signify that the imbalance was environmentally determined, though the tendency might be innate?

Perhaps. One thing is sure. Whatever the impetus, it is the left-hander and his spatial ability that yield to pressure, then present themselves to statistical scrutiny. We are still looking for a comparable group of right-handers who reveal a corresponding hemispherically lopsided superiority of spatial over verbal talent. For that matter, Levy is still looking for a group of left-handers that do. (She thinks she may have found it in a study of predominantly left-handed architects. Unfortunately, however, the researcher who tested them ignored the verbal factor.)

Levy would insist that her Cal Tech lefties were different, but not necessarily inferior. But other researchers would oppose her corollary contention that left-handers in general are not inferior neurologically, even when they are demonstrably different.

Indeed, according to a wealth of accumulated experimental evidence, left-handers by and large seldom outperform their dextral brothers and sisters on *any* motor or sensory task—except, perhaps, playing baseball or tennis (where their very difference gives them an initial competitive edge) and seeing under water (possibly because they may be better in touch with the more abundant visual receptors of their non-language hemisphere).

Right-handers, in contrast, usually prevail in a host of across-the-board measures designed to demonstrate the soundness, stability, sensitivity, functional efficiency, perceptual keenness, and all-round high-caliber performance of their central nervous systems.

They integrate visual and auditory stimuli better and respond to brightness in both visual fields with a symmetry left-handers in general cannot hope to match. They make color distinctions with greater acuity and color matchings with greater speed, even when efforts are made to thwart them with fast shuffles and sudden, unexpected maskings. In addition, their lateral eye movement is more consistently telling—and consequently a more reliable predictor of scholastic aptitude—than that of the mercurial left-hander. Their tactile perceptions of such divergent qualities as size and pain are more closely related in either hand, as well. They are also, on the average, better at *both* verbal and tactile/spatial tasks. As children, Martha Bridge Denckla of Columbia University found, their motor responses on coordination tests are superior—in the hand opposite the hemisphere controlling for that speciality.

And finally, for what it may mean, they are even more susceptible to hypnosis.

Taken as a whole, then, the left-hander is manifestly inferior from almost every neurological standpoint. But given the fact that while some of them are probably brain-damaged, many more are not, perhaps that is just the point: Left-handers should never be taken as a whole. In neurosurgeon Joseph Bogen's words, "Right-handers are a bunch of chocolate soldiers. If you've seen one, you've seen 'em all. But left-handers are something else again."[15]

What happens, say, if we separate those who are left-handed on many tasks from those left-handed on a few, divide the "strong" left-handers from the "weak"?

In instances where this has been done, a distinctly different pattern emerges. In facial recognition, in verbal/spatial distinctions, in visual and auditory perception—*strong left-handers prove as accomplished as strong right-handers.* Only weak left-handers lag behind—so far behind they drag the entire left-hand population down below the right.

Who are the strong left-handers, the weak left-handers? How are we to tell them apart? At what cutoff point in handedness testing can the one be said with confidence to end and the other begin? Is either related to family history?

In at least one visual discrimination test where careful family backgrounds were compiled, the group that performed best were the right-handers with *no family history of left-handedness.* Needless to say, the greater degree of left-handedness, the poorer the performance. But whether the enduring neurological deficits can be split away and laid at the doorstep of inheritance—a deficit either transmitted directly or indirectly by the genes or by something as potentially influential as a legacy or injuriously defective birth canals—remains to be seen.

And what, finally, of that old bugaboo, criteria? Shall we define handedness primarily in terms of skill or preference, strength or cunning, consistency or—prejudicial word—dexterity?

Possibly, as we shall now see, Jerre Levy has the answer.

174

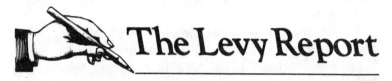

The Levy Report

15

Several years ago, Jerre Levy noticed a curious hand anomaly in the most unlikely place for a researcher to look: her husband. He was right-handed, but he wrote with his wrist hooked over the paper, the pencil pointing toward the bottom of the page. Such a style is common to left-handers, of course, but Levy could not recall ever seeing a right-hander use it.

Once sensitized, however, she began, over the next few years, to see more and more of them—a phenomenon of focused attention that may be just as important as what she found. After all, scientists were certain the prehistoric fish coelacanth was extinct until they pulled up a living specimen, then discovered it was a diet staple all around the Indian ocean.

Levy had always assumed the psychological literature was correct, that such hooking in left-handers was a kind of peripheral compensation to offset the left-to-right, against-their-grain flow of Western writing. That this explanation could equally hold for hooking right-handers, far fewer though they were, struck her as a dubious proposition. It became, in her words, "patently false" when she took a long look at hand-writing in Israel. There, people write "backward," that is to say, from right to left. And here again, left-handers hooked in large numbers, right-handers only rarely.

Since it obviously had nothing to do with the direction of writing, Levy decided hooking must in some way reflect brain organization. "I said, 'gee, that's funny, left-handers falling into two classes, those who write this way and those who write that way,'" she remembers.

It was especially exciting, not to mention methodologically neat, in the light of the well-established fact that left-handers could have language in either hemisphere. "So," says Levy, "I postulated that left-handers who write with their hand hooked had language in the left side of the brain, and left-handers who wrote in the uninverted fashion, the nonhookers, had language in the *right* side of the brain.

"In other words, they were a mirror image of the normal right-hander. Their contralateral control for language came from the right hemisphere to the left hand, instead of from the left hemisphere to the right hand."

Hookers, in contrast, expressed the same-side brain-to-hand control for language that she and Nagylaki had postulated in their genetic model. That control could be either left-side or right-side, as both kinds of hookers demonstrated.

Farfetched as their critics had originally found such an idea, Levy saw further dramatic evidence for it every day, in a pickled nervous system at the University of Pennsylva-

176

nia neurology department. It was entirely split into two unconnected halves, yet fully matured. There were no decussations, no crossing fibers at all. Yet surely its owner had lived and died a reasonably functioning human being!

In collaboration with psychologist Marylou Reid, Levy set out to prove her thesis with a pair of visual tests that would determine the direction of brain lateralization in a group of seventy-three university volunteers. They included two dozen normal right-handers, two dozen left-handers who hooked in handwriting and two dozen who didn't, as well as a solitary right-hand-hooking coed. All groups were divided equally by sex.

One of the tests was designed to measure the spatial ability of their brains, the other the verbal, each of which is thought usually to reside in a separate hemisphere. Each subject was asked to fix his or her eyes on a point straight ahead. Spatial or verbal information was flashed in random sequence to one or the other visual field and its controlling hemisphere, too fast for eye movements to shift the stimulus to the other side—a cooperative strategy the normal, healthy brain is believed to pursue on most of life's tasks. One test required them to identify and pronounce nonsense words, the other to locate the position of rapidly flashed dots by touching a tactile matrix.

Normal right-handers typically do better on the verbal test in their right visual fields, of course, because language is specialized to the left hemisphere. Conversely, they are better in their left visual fields on the dot-location test because the right hemisphere is more adept at spatial mapping.

Since this division is about as well established in neurophysiology as anything, Levy and Reid refined their two tests until they yielded exactly those results in right-

177

handers almost one hundred percent of the time. Then, using that as their baseline for comparison, they turned a probing eye on the anomalies—both kinds of left-handers and the one hooking right-hander.

If Levy's thinking was correct, the hooking right-hander should perform exactly opposite the normal right-handers, which is to say, like the non-hooking left-handers. She should show a left-visual-field superiority for the word test if her language were centered in the right hemisphere, on the same side as her preferred hand.

And the left-handers? The hookers, Levy predicted, would perform exactly opposite the nonhookers, which is to say, like the nonhooking right-handers. Each group, in short, hookers and nonhookers, would mirror-image each other.

As it happens, Levy and Reid found exactly that. It was in fact, as Levy says, the first time "somebody has been able to predict ahead of time what the direction of brain lateralization in the left-hander was going to be."

But the researchers found much more, a lot of it hardly reconcilable with what we have traditionally come to believe about brain organization. Unlike her earlier study group of left-handers in general at Cal Tech, the nonhooking left-handers proved just as well lateralized in their abilities as right-handers.

"They just went off in opposite directions," she stresses. "They are just as laterally differentiated as most right-handers. If you took a right-hander and set him in front of a mirror, his reflected image would be this group of nonhooking left-handers."

The *hooking* left-handers displayed a very small degree of lateral differentiation between their hemispheres—so little, in fact, that it prompted Levy to conclude that the Cal

178

Tech discrepancy "specifically pertains to the hooking left-handers, those who have language in the left side of the brain." That may have been why several other researchers had failed to replicate Levy's results: Their mix of hooking and nonhooking left-handers had been different.

Somewhat surprisingly, there was little else in the data to distinguish the two, dramatically different, kinds of left-handedness from each other. A preliminary questionnaire on which hand the subjects used for what betrayed no telling contrasts. Levy decided such a written technique simply wasn't sensitive enough:

"I think if I had measured actual skills, the nonhooking left-hander would have shown a bigger left-hand superiority over his right, just as the normal right-hander shows a big right-hand superiority over his left.

"But I'm only guessing."

Nor was family the factor some might have suspected. Not surprisingly, both groups of left-handers had more sinistrals in their family than did right-handers. But surprisingly, neither had markedly more as a group than the other. "I thought at first that the hooking left-handers were the ones with brain damage, because they had such a small degree of lateral differentiation," Levy admits. "But under that hypothesis you would expect they wouldn't have as many left-handed family members. Yet they did.

"It could be, of course, that some of them *are* brain-damaged, and so are their family members. Maybe it has something to do with deficient birth canals in the mothers. Maybe what's really running in these families is difficult births."

As for their scores, Levy and Reid found them amazingly mixed. On the average, hooking left-handers did poorer than the other two groups, but the exceptions were even

179

more interesting. On the dot location test, eight out of the twelve hooking males did worse than every single male right-hander. Only one was even in the same range. But even more bizarre, *three of the other four outperformed every single right-hander by an astonishing amount.*

Marvels Levy, "I mean, their performance was so high it was inconceivable to me how they were doing it." Even when she reduced exposure time and introduced masking bits of visual stimuli to push them to their limits, their skill never faltered.

"I couldn't even *see* a dot under those conditions," she remembers. "Literally, I couldn't see one, much less specify its location."

For the mirror-image left-handers—the nonhookers with language in their right hemispheres—Levy concluded that the possibility of brain damage was out of the question. Their relative performance was just too high and consistent.

But hooking left-handers, particularly males, being either very good or very bad and consequently bracketing all their right-handed counterparts, were something else again. Clearly the best of them were miles beyond the taint of such suspicion. As Levy remarks, "If they're brain-damaged, they're the biggest tragedy in the world because, even so, they outperform everybody. Just imagine what they'd be like if they weren't!"

But those at the bottom of the scale suggest some left-handedness may indeed be pathological, the result of trauma. In their pretest trials to screen out possible cerebral injury, Levy and Reid eliminated four subjects who displayed response patterns which might be expected with brain damage.

Although all were university students doing passing work, they alone of the seventy-seven original subjects

180

failed to demonstrate absolutely symmetrical thresholds for a simple dot detection by the visual fields of both hemispheres.

Rather, reports Levy, they showed "a whopping asymmetry" requiring at least twice as much exposure time to one hemisphere as the other. In sum, all had a hemisphere, either one or the other, that was manifestly defective in the simple visual perception.

Their handedness? One was a normal right-hander, the other three hooking left-handers. The preponderance of hooking left-handers even in such a small sample, Levy believes, "does suggest that something funny is going on. It's quite possible that pathological left-handers tend to be left-hookers. But that doesn't necessarily mean that all left-hookers are pathological.

"It does suggest that if you're going to look for pathological left-handers, you're more likely to find them here than anywhere."

The final anomaly—and ultimately the most provocative in its implications—was the lone hooking right-hander. As predicted, she showed a left-hemisphere superiority on dot location and a right-hemisphere superiority on the word test, exactly opposite the normal right-hander. True to Levy's model, she demonstrated language and handedness on the same side, suggesting ipsilateral (same side) control mirror-imaging that of the hooking left-hander.

So far so good. But when Levy compared her performance to that of the other right-handers, she got her first shock. She found that although the girl did extremely well on dot location, *she scored lower verbally than all other seventy-two subjects, men and women alike.*

Something was wrong here. Women, after all, historically tend to score better verbally on the average than men. Even if her brain were as poorly lateralized as that of the hooking left-hander, the likelihood of her being outscored by all the non-hooking right-handed males in the test group—much less the poorly lateralized hooking left-handed males—was exceedingly slim. In view of her high spatial score, it could hardly be that her brain was just inferior. What could be the explanation?

Almost by serendipity Levy stumbled onto the solution, one she concedes is tentative and suggests is "the strangest thing in the world." It appeared when she sat down to examine differences in the comparative performance of all volunteers in the group by sex.

In the group of normal right-handers, the males did better on dot location than on words, the females better on words than on dot location, as expected. The same held true, she found, for the hooking left-handers. Again, there was nothing unforeseen about that. Their brains, after all, were organized the same, with language in the left hemisphere, spatial relations in the right. Only their hand control—ipsilateral or same-side instead of contralateral or opposite-side—differed.

But then Levy looked at her nonhooking, or mirror-image, left-handers and got another shock. *Their performance was exactly reversed: The males did better on verbal than spatial, the females better on spatial than verbal!*

"This was completely at odds with the psychological literature," she recalls. "It says females show a deficiency on spatial, males a deficiency on verbal. That was true for a majority of my subjects, namely right-handers and the hooking left-handers. But it obviously wasn't true for those in whom the site of language was reversed and wound up in the right hemisphere: the nonhooking left-hander and my one hooking right-hander.

"Here you got a reversal of the normal sex pattern. The males were better in verbal, the females better on spatial."

Consistent with these results was the fact that Levy's right-hooking husband was very much higher on verbal than on spatial IQ. In collaboration with Raquel and Ruben Gur, Levy next gave standardized paper-and-pencil tests to a manually mixed group of college girls. The girls, in turn, likewise nailed down her thesis. The normal right-handers did better verbally, and so did the hooking left-handers. But the nonhooking left-handers—those with language in the right hemisphere—did better spatially.

"What this is suggesting is something so strange I don't know what to make of it," Levy says today. "In every single group, *whatever females are better on, the males are better on the opposite.* In females the functions of the *left* side of the brain are enhanced relative to those on the right, regardless of *what* the left hemisphere programs.

"If you've got language in your left hemisphere and you're a female, you're going to be better on language than on spatial functions. But if you've got spatial functions in the left hemisphere and you're female, you're going to be better on spatial functions."

On the other hand, in males, Levy found, the *right* hemisphere's performance is enhanced relative to the left's, regardless of *what* the right hemisphere programs: "In other words, if you've got spatial abilities in your right hemisphere and you're male, you're going to be better on spatial tasks than on language.

"But if you've got language in your right hemisphere and you're male, you're going to be better on verbal functions."

Levy's colleague, Marylou Reid, has since determined that in children the specialities of the left hemisphere develop first in girls, the specialities of the right first in boys—regardless of *what's* there.

As Levy says: "For years everybody's been talking, my-

183

self included, about the idea that verbal functions are enhanced in females and spatial functions enhanced in males. But that doesn't describe my data. What describes my data is that it's not the function that's enhanced, it's the *hemisphere*—left in females, right in males.''

Extraordinary as they appear, Levy's findings are not beyond question. When mentioned in a recent publication, they drew pragmatic fire from hooking left-handers, who protested that there was nothing natural about their propensity at all. They hooked, they said, because their teachers had made them slant their paper in the wrong direction (like right-handers), because the rings of looseleaf or spiral notebooks got in their way, or because they wanted to see what they had written.

These explanations, of course, fail to account for the noninverted left-handers, who presumably overcame their teachers, notebooks, and curiosity about the sentence in progress, to write as they damn well pleased. But the hooking-nonhooking split is not without dispute from other quarters.

One woman I know, for instance, told me she was originally a hooking left-hander, but had been changed by her father, who had always written left-handedly without hooking. Since a change of hands is not unusual (from left to right, naturally), a change of style with the same hand would not be all that difficult either—although it does raise the specter of transcallosal control which Levy concedes as a possibility but finds inelegant except under pressure.

Then again, another left-handed acquaintance of mine, a teenage girl, writes with her hand hooked but *draws* in the noninverted manner. Since the ability to draw would normally be controlled by the visual-spatial program of her right hemisphere, such a distinction makes eminent sense—

184

in theory. But does this mean, then, as it must, that Levy's noninverted left-handers would hook in drawing? None of them mentioned it. And if not, how would their visual-spatial left hemisphere communicate with and control their left hands without the same kind of unaesthetic traffic across the commissures that Levy finds stupid?

Levy classifies such anomalies as "ambiguous" and confesses, "I shall have to look at them someday."

One thing she may have to look at earlier is the intriguing failure of at least one handedness researcher in replicating her results. Using an EEG and evoked potentials to determine which hemisphere was switched on when the left-handers performed, Jeannine Herron of San Francisco's Langley Porter Neuropsychiatric Institute was unable to find any strong, consistent indication of such same-side control.

Finally, as noted in an earlier chapter, Yakovlev found that his four allegedly left-handed specimens had *the same left-to-right crossing of preponderant nerve fibers that characterized the right-handers*. That raises some question about the neurological basis for Levy's conclusions regarding crossed versus same-side control of handedness. How can she claim too *few* crossing fibers are significant while too *many* are not necessarily?

Levy is undaunted. In the light of her highly consistent experimental results, she sees no reason for supposing, *without proof,* that the right-of-way of the majority of these motor fibers mitigates against her theory when the *size* of the lower crossing tracts might tell a different story.

Barring further exposure of the intact spinal cord in a significant sample of postmortem specimens and a definitive tracing of its entire wiring plan, she sticks to her empirical guns.

Her data, Levy believes, indicate the existence of at least *seven different kinds* of basic brain organization, perhaps eight if you count the hooking right-hander, whose single set of scores is nothing to generalize about

The overwhelming majority of people is made up of male right-handers, male mirror-image (noninverted) left-handers, female right-handers, and female mirror-image left-handers—each with a different alignment of hemispheres. These Levy calls "cognitive generalists." Though their hemispheres are enhanced differentially by sex, they are, she believes, "pretty good in just about everything."

The minority, in turn, is made up of hooking left-handers (and probably hooking right-handers) of both sexes. Because their hemispheres are poorly lateralized, Levy is convinced, from the patterns of their scores, that the functions of each merge to create three different kinds of performers. Two of them she calls "cognitive specialists." She says, "They tend to be very good at one set of abilities and relatively depressed in the other." As the definition implies, they are those whose spatial functions invade and dominate the language side, and those whose language functions invade and dominate the spatial side—regardless, perhaps, of which sex, which hand, or which side is which.

The third category where lateralization breaks down and overlap occurs is that in which the function of *either* side invades and diminishes the other, with the effect that *both* kinds of ability are depressed.

"What I'm guessing right now is that these incompletely lateralized people are the result of congenital reasons," says Levy, "possibly genetic. But the form it takes doesn't seem to be under control of that same gene. What's specialized is that you're going to be incompletely lateralized. The

186

form it takes will be determined by other factors, possibly levels of fetal hormones, genes occuring at other places—all kinds of things. I need more data on this, but that's my tentative interpretation.

"Isn't that crazy?"[1]

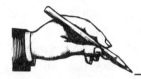

Epilogue

Crazy it is, but that's it. For all we know, statistics do tell the truth: There really are, as Domhoff points out, "left (permissive) epochs"[1] in which left-handedness increases, and wars and depressions in which sinistrality is more than *seven times* as frequent as normal—in college graduates, at least. We might as well attribute the trait to sociological uncertainty and be done with it—or, as Domhoff does, couple it to hair length as "good indicators of 'left' and 'right' historical periods, or 'matrist' and 'patrist' [mother and father] periods."[2]

For even if Jerre Levy is correct, her findings help us left-handers little. Lacking her sophisticated testing equipment, we whose writing was switched in childhood will never know which of these many ways our brain is wired, much less what we might do about it. Those who still write left-handedly, for that matter, scarcely stand to profit from such knowledge in a practical way, either. Like the rest of us, they are what they are, perform as they do, and knowing their brains are organized for visual skills better than verbal ones will not turn an average English teacher into a crack auto mechanic—unless, perhaps, he already leans in that direction. (Mercifully, it will not turn a brilliant English teacher into a humdrum mechanic either, which may be more than we can say for many of the human-potential therapies and practices now sweeping the country.)

The best we can hope for is that such knowledge will work itself into the school system and bring about greater latitude there, both in teaching techniques and the skills we value. That, really, is the most important thing we are talking about. Recent discoveries about handedness, inconclusive as they may be, argue—if argument is necessary—for an ever-deepening appreciation of human diversity. As Levy says:

"As soon as we left the jungle and went out onto the savanna, we *had* to be a social species. I think there was a biological basis for this specialization, different kinds of [genes] in different frequencies for different kinds of cognitive structures: not only the fully lateralized generalizers, but the specialists as well, your super mapmakers, your super conceptualizers, or whatever.

"If I'm right, if it turns out that females have the left side of their brains enhanced and males the right, then these variations would simply bring in more different varieties of brain organization.

"The result of such a 'balanced polymorphism,' as I call mankind, has all kinds of sociological implications, foremost that we're crazy as a species if we try to push everybody through the same cookie mold—that we're *biological-*

ly meant to be diverse, and that such diversity is helpful to all of us."[3]

If Levy is right, if the human race is gifted with several distinct types of "wiring plans" for its brain, the net result will be nothing so parochial as to "give the game to the neurologists," as a psychologist friend of mine narrowly laments. The game is there to be played by *everybody,* not just each individual himself as he attempts somewhat to shape his own destiny, but to everyone in all fields that even remotely depend on the function, development, education, and reward of the human brain.

As psychobiologist Roger Sperry of the California Institute of Technology writes so succinctly, "differential balance and loading between these right and left hemispheric faculties . . . could make for quite a spectrum of individual variations in the structure of human intellect—from the mechanical or artistic geniuses on the one hand who can hardly express themselves in writing or speech, to the highly articulate individuals at the other extreme who think almost entirely in verbal terms."[4]

Left-handers, of course, need not apply. They are already included by the marvelous vagaries of their very nature. Remember Leonardo.

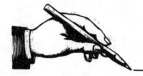 # Notes

PROLOGUE

1. Van Buren, "Soft in the Heart," p. 46.

CHAPTER 1

1. Personal communication.
2. Barsley, *Left-Handed People*, pp. 129–30.
3. Gardner, *The Ambidextrous Universe*, p. 82.

CHAPTER 2

1. The Bible, King James Version, Matthew 6:3.
2. *Ibid.*, Matthew 25:32–41.
3. *Ibid.*, Jonah 4: 11.

4. Barsley, *op. cit.*, p. 99.
5. The Bible, King James Version, Judges 20: 16.
6. Yakovlev, "Telokinesis and Handedness," p. 21.
7. Hécaen and de Ajuriaguerra, *Left-Handedness*, p. 125.
8. *Ibid.*
9. Whitehead, Encyclopaedia Britannica, 1974, Vol. 14, p. 538.
10. Hécaen and de Ajuriaguerra, *Left-Handedness*, p. 125.
11. *Ibid.*, p. 121.
12. Domhoff, "But Why Do They Sit on the King's Right in the First Place?" pp. 588–89.
13. *Ibid.*, p. 589.
14. C. J. Jung, *Man and His Symbols* (Garden City, New York: Doubleday & Co., 1964), p. 215.

CHAPTER 3

1. Hertz, *Death and the Right Hand*, p. 19.
2. *Ibid.*, p. 98.
3. *Ibid.*, p. 106.
4. *Ibid.*, p. 104.
5. *Ibid.*
6. *Ibid.*, p. 107.
7. *Ibid.*
8. *Ibid.*, p. 97.
9. *Ibid.*, p. 105.
10. *Ibid.*, p. 108.
11. *Ibid.*
12. De Kay, *The Left-Handed Book*, p. 44.
13. Faron, "Symbolic Values Among the Mapuche," p. 1156.
14. Hertz, *op. cit.*, p. 112.
15. *Ibid.*, pp. 105–6.
16. *Ibid.*, p. 106.
17. *Ibid.*
18. *Ibid.*
19. *Ibid.*, p. 103.
20. *Ibid.*, p. 110.

21. *Ibid.*, p. 112.
22. *Ibid.*
23. *Ibid.*, p. 110.
24. *Ibid.* p. 98.
25. Domhoff, *op cit.*, p. 594.
26. Hertz, *op. cit.*, p. 113.

CHAPTER 4

1. Levy, "Psychobiological Implications of Bilateral Asymmetry," p. 121.
2. *Ibid.*
3. *Ibid.*
4. Blau, *The Master Hand*, p. 60.
5. *Ibid.*, p. 53.
6. *Ibid.*, p. 61.
7. *Ibid.*
8. *Ibid.*
9. *Ibid.*, p. 64.
10. Hecaen and de Ajuriaguerra, *Left-Handedness*, p. 130.
11. Blau, *The Master Hand*, p. 32.

CHAPTER 5

1. Gardner, *The Ambidextrous Universe*, p. 43.

CHAPTER 6

1. Gardner, *The Ambidextrous Universe*, p. 99.
2. *Ibid.*, p. 102.
3. *Ibid.*, p. 101.
4. *Ibid.*, p. 102.
5. *Ibid.*, p. 140.
6. *Ibid.*, p. 141.

CHAPTER 7

1. Gardner, "Can Time Go Backward?" p. 2
2. *Ibid.*
3. *Ibid.*, p. 3.
4. *Ibid.*
5. Gardner, *The Ambidextrous Universe*, p. 188.
6. *Ibid.*, p. 209.
7. *Ibid.*, p. 191.
8. Wigner, "Violations of Symmetry in Physics," p. 35. (Italics added.)

CHAPTER 8

1. Gardner, *The Ambidextrous Universe*, p. 60.
2. *Ibid.*, p. 70.
3. Nagylaki and Levy, "The Sound of One Paw Clapping Isn't Sound," p. 279.
4. *Ibid.*
5. *Ibid.*, p. 287.

CHAPTER 9

1. Yakovlev, "Telokinesis and Handedness," p. 22.
2. *Ibid.*, p. 23.
3. Yakovlev, "A Proposed Definition of the Limbic System," p. 21.
4. Gardner, *The Ambidextrous Universe*, p. 218.
5. *Ibid.*, p. 219.
6. *Ibid.*
7. *Ibid.*
8. Personal communication.
9. *Ibid.*
10. *Ibid.*

11. *Ibid.*
12. Yakovlev, "A Proposed Definition of the Limbic System," p. 259.
13. *Ibid.,* p. 269.
14. *Ibid.*
15. *Ibid.,* p. 259.
16. Yakovlev, "Telokinesis and Handedness," p. 27.
17. Yakovlev, "A Proposed Definition of the Limbic System," p. 272.
18. Yakovlev, "Telokinesis and Handedness," p. 28.
19. *Ibid.,* p. 29.

CHAPTER 10

1. Personal interview.
2. Yakovlev and Rakic, "Decussation of Bulbar Pyramids and Distribution of Pyramidal Tracts," p. 366.
3. Yakovlev, "A Proposed Definition of the Limbic System," p. 275.
4. *Ibid.*
5. Turkewitz and Creighton, "Lateral Differential of Head Posture," pp. 85–86.
6. Brown, *New Mind, New Body,* p. 102.
7. Friedlander, "Some Aspects of Eyedness," p. 357.

CHAPTER 11

1. Levy, "Psychobiological Implications of Bilateral Asymmetry," p. 167.
2. Bogen, "Other Side of the Brain, II," p. 156.
3. Levy, *Evolution of the Nervous System,* pp. 60–71.
4. Broca, in Blau, *The Master Hand,* p. 14.
5. Broca, in Hertz, *Death and the Right Hand,* p. 90.
6. Bird, "Leboyer Follow-Up," p. 14.
7. *Ibid.*

CHAPTER 12

1. Blau, *The Master Hand,* p. 44.
2. *Ibid.*
3. *Ibid.*
4. *Ibid.*
5. Corballis and Morgan, "On the Biological Basis of Human Laterality," p. 19.
6. Levy, personal communication.
7. *Ibid.*
8. Corballis and Morgan, op. cit., p. 20.
9. *Ibid.,* p. 21.
10. *Ibid.,* p. 22.
11. Annett, "The Distribution of Manual Asymmetry," p. 357.
12. *Ibid.*
13. Corballis and Morgan, *op. cit.,* p. 24.
14. Corballis and Beale, "On Telling Left from Right," p. 96.
15. *Ibid.,* p. 100.
16. *Ibid.*
17. Corballis and Morgan, *op. cit.,* p. 9.
18. *Ibid.,* p. 10.
19. *Ibid.,* Abstract.
20. Levy, personal communication.
21. Corballis and Morgan, *op. cit.,* p. 30.
22. Satz, "Pathological Left-Handedness," p. 122.

CHAPTER 13

1. Blau, *The Master Hand.*
2. Oldfield, "The Assessment and Analysis of Handedness," p. 101.
3. *Ibid.,* p. 104.
4. *Ibid.*
5. Oldfield, *op. cit.,* p. 99.
6. Mecklin, personal communication.

CHAPTER 14

1. De Kay, "The Lobal Society of Southpaws," p. 196.
2. *Ibid.*
3. Barsley, *Left-Handed People,* p. 131.
4. De Kay, "Southpaws," p. 196.
5. *Ibid.*
6. Bryngelson, in Lo Bello, "Are Left-Handers All Right?" 83.
7. *Ibid.*
8. Blau, in Trotter, "Sinister Psychology," p. 221.
9. *Ibid.*
10. Bell, "Our President, the Southpaw," p. 4.
11. Cavanaugh, "The One-Armed Wonder," p. 58.
12. Herron, "Southpaws—How Different Are They?" p. 53.
13. Bakan, "Left-Handedness and Alcoholism," p. 514.
14. Clarke, "The World of the Dyslexic Child," p. 60.
15. Bogen, "Mind as Healer, Mind as Slayer," Oct. 31, 1975.

CHAPTER 15

All quotes in this chapter are from personal communication with Levy.

EPILOGUE

1. Domhoff, "But Why Do They Sit on the King's Right?" p. 594.
2. *Ibid.*, p. 596.
3. Levy, personal communication.
4. Sperry, "Lateral Specialization of Cerebral Function," p. 221.

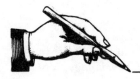

Bibliography

BOOKS

BARSLEY, MICHAEL. *Left-Handed People*. North Hollywood: Wilshire Book Company, 1976.

BLAU, ABRAM. *The Master Hand*. American Orthopsychiatric Association, 1946.

BROWN, B. *New Mind, New Body*. New York: Harper & Row, 1974.

DE KAY, JAMES T. *The Left-Handed Book*. New York: M. Evans & Company, Inc., 1966

GARDNER, MARTIN. *The Ambidextrous Universe*. New York: The New American Library, 1969.

HÉCAEN, HENRY, and DE AJURIAGUERRA, JULIAN. *Left-Handedness: Manual Superority and Cerebral Dominance*. Grune & Stratton, 1964.

HERTZ, ROBERT. *Death and the Right Hand*. New York: The Free Press, 1960.

SARNAT, HARVEY B. and NETSKY, MARTIN G. *Evolution of the Nervous System.* New York: Oxford University Press, 1974.

SYMPOSIUM

BOGEN, JOSEPH E. "Mind as Healer, Mind as Slayer," University of California, Berkeley, Oct. 31 to Nov. 2, 1975.

ARTICLES

ANNETT, MARIAN. "A Classification of Hand Preference by Association Analysis." *British Journal of Psychology,* Vol. 61, No. 3, 1970.

ANNETT, MARIAN. "The Distribution of Manual Asymmetry." *British Journal of Psychology,* Vol. 63, No. 3, 1972.

ANNETT, MARIAN. "The Growth of Manual Preference and Speed." *British Journal of Psychology,* Vol. 61, No. 2, 1970.

ANNETT, MARIAN. "Handedness in the Children of Two Left-Handed Parents." *British Journal of Psychology,* Vol. 65, No. 1, 1974.

ANNETT, MARIAN, HUDSON, P. J. W., and TURNER, ANN. "The Reliability of Differences Between the Hands in Motor Skills." *Neuropsychologia,* Vol. 12, October, 1974.

BAKAN, PAUL. "Left-Handedness and Alcoholism." *Perceptual and Motor Skills,* Vol. 36, April, 1973.

BAKAN, PAUL. "Right-Left Discrimination and Brain Lateralization (Sex Differences)." *Archives of Neurology,* Vol. 30, April, 1974.

BARNSLEY, ROGER H., and RABINOVITCH, SAM. "Handedness: Proficiency Versus Stated Preference." *Perceptual and Motor Skills,* Vol. 30, April, 1970.

BELL, JIM. "Our President the Southpaw." *San Francisco Examiner and Chronicle,* October 20, 1974.

BIRD, CHRISTOPHER. "Leboyer Follow-up." *New Age Journal,* February, 1975.

BOGEN, JOSEPH E. "The Other Side of the Brain—II: An Appositional Mind." *Bulletin of the Los Angeles Neurological Socïety*, July, 1969.

BUTLER, S. R., and GLASS, A. "Asymmetries in the CNV Over Left and Right Hemispheres While Subjects Await Numeric Information." *Biological Psychology*, 2, 1974.

CAVANAUGH, JACK. "The One-Armed Wonder," *True* magazine, November, 1975.

CERNACEK, J., and PODIVINSKY, F. "Ontogenesis of Handedness and Somatosensory Cortical Response." *Neuropsychologia*, Vol. 9, June, 1971.

CHANG, K. S. F., HSU, F. K., CHAN, S. T., and CHAN, Y. B. "Scrotal Asymmetry and Handedness." *Journal of Anatomy*, Vol. 94, September, 1960.

CLARKE, LOUISE. "The World of the Dyslexic Child." *Family Health*, October, 1974.

COLE, J. "Laterality in the Use of the Hand, Foot and Eye in Monkeys." *Journal of Comparative Physiology and Psychology*, Vol. 50, 1957.

COLLINS, ROBERT L. "When Left-Handed Mice Live in Right-Handed Worlds." *Science*, January 17, 1975.

CORBALLIS, MICHAEL C., and BEALE, IVAN L. "On Telling Left from Right." *Scientific American*, March, 1971.

CORBALLIS, MICHAEL C., and MORGAN, MICHAEL J. "On the Biological Basis of Human Laterality." Courtesy of the authors and as yet unpublished.

DAVIDOFF, J. B. "Hemispheric Differences in the Perception of Lightness." *Neuropsychologia*, Vol. 13, January, 1975.

DEE, H. L. "Auditory Asymmetry and Strength of Manual Preference." *Cortex*, September, 1971.

DE KAY, JAMES T. "The Lobal Society of Southpaws." *Horizon*, Summer, 1974.

DENCKLA, MARTHA BRIDGE. "Development of Motor Co-Ordination in Normal Children." *Developmental Medicine and Child Neurology*, Vol. 16, 1974.

DEVANNA, JAN. "The Only Liberation Movement That's Left." *North Jersey Herald-News* Magazine, March 15, 1975.

DIMOND, STUART, and BEAUMONT, GRAHAM. "Hemisphere

Function and Color Naming." *Journal of Experimental Psychology*, Vol. 96, No. 1, 1972.

DOMHOFF, G. WILLIAM. "But Why Do They Sit on the King's Right in the First Place?" *Psychoanalytic Review*, Winter, 1969-1970.

ENGLUND, STEVEN. "Birth Without Violence." *The New York Times Magazine*, December 8, 1974.

FAGIN-DUBIN, L. "Lateral Dominance and Development of Cerebral Specialization." *Cortex*, March, 1974.

FARON, LOUIS C. "Symbolic Values and the Integration of Society Among the Mapuche of Chile." *American Anthropologist*, Vol. 64, 1972.

FINN, JANE A., and NEURINGER, CHARLES. "Left-Handedness: A Study of Its Relation to Opposition." *Journal of Projective Techniques and Personality Assessment*, Vol. 32, No. 1, 1968.

FRIEDLANDER, WALTER J. "Some Aspects of Eyedness." *Cortex*, December 7, 1972.

FROST, BETTY. "Dr. Leboyer Talks About Non-Violent Childbirth." San Rafael, California: *Independent Journal*, December 3, 1975.

GARDNER, MARTIN. "Can Time Go Backward?" *Scientific American*, January, 1967.

GILBERT, CHRISTOPHER. "Strength of Left-Handedness and Facial Recognition Ability." *Cortex*, January, 1973.

GUR, RUBIN C., and RAQUEL E. "Handedness, Sex, and Eyedness as Moderating Variables in the Relation Between Hypnotic Susceptibility and Functional Brain Asymmetry." *Journal of Abnormal Psychology*, Vol. 83, No. 6, 1974.

HAMMER, MADELINE, and TURKEWITZ, GERALD. "A Sensory Basis for the Lateral Difference in the Newborn Infant's Response to Somesthetic Stimulation." *Journal of Experimental Child Psychology*, Vol. 18, October, 1974.

HASLAM, DIANA R. "Lateral Dominance in the Perception of Size and of Pain." *British Journal of Experimental Psychology*, Vol. 22, August, 1970.

HÉCAEN, H., and SAUGUET, J. "Cerebral Dominance in Left-Handed Subjects." *Cortex*, March, 1971.

HECK, THOMAS. "The Sex Habit Nobody Talks About." *True* Magazine, December, 1975.

HERRON, JEANNINE. "Southpaws—How Different Are They?" *Psychology Today*, March, 1976.

HICKOK, ANDRÉE. "Westporter Comes to the Aid of Frustrated Lefties." Bridgeport *Sunday Post*, May 27, 1973.

HINES, DAVID, and SATZ, PAUL. "Cross-Modal Asymmetries in Perception Related to Asymmetry in Cerebral Function." *Neuropsychologia*, Vol. 12, March, 1974.

HORN, JACK. "The Hand Is Faster Than the Eye, Especially If You Read Backwards." News Line. *Psychology Today*, November, 1975.

JONES, R. K., "Observations on Stammering After Localized Cerebral Injury." *Journal of Neurology, Neurosurgery and Psychiatry*, Vol. 29, 1966.

KATZ, DOLORES. "By Right We Should Have More Lefties." San Francisco *Sunday Examiner and Chronicle*, June 1, 1975.

KELLER, JAMES F., CROAKE, JAMES W., and RIESENMAN, CAROLYN. "Relationships Among Handedness, Intelligence, Sex and Reading Achievement of School Age Children." *Perceptual and Motor Skills*, Vol. 37, August, 1973.

KIMURA, DOREEN, and VANDERWOLF, C. H. "The Relation Between Hand Preference and the Performance of Individual Finger Movements by Left and Right Hands." *Brain*, Vol. 93, 1970.

KINSBOURNE, MARCEL. "Eye and Head Turning Indicates Cerebral Lateralization." *Science*, May 5, 1972.

KUTAS, MARTA, and DONCHIN, EMANUEL. "Studies of Squeezing: Handedness, Responding Hand, Response Force, and Asymmetry of Readiness Potential." *Science*, November 8, 1974.

LASS, NORMAN J., KOTCHEK, CYNTHIA L., and DEEM, JODELLE F. "Oral Two-Point Discrimination: Further Evidence of Asymmetry on Right and Left Sides of Selected Oral Structures." *Perceptual and Motor Skills,* Vol. 35, August, 1972.

LEVITAN, IRWIN B., RAMIREZ, GALO, and MUSHYNSKI, WALTER E. "Amino Acid Incorporation in the Brains of Rats Trained to Use the Non-Preferred Paw in Retrieving Food." *Brain Research,* Vol. 47, 1972.

LEVY, JERRE. "Psychobiological Implications of Bilateral Asymmetry." *Hemisphere Function in the Human Brain.* Dimond, S., and Beaumont, J. G., editors. London: Paul Elek, Ltd., 1974.

LO BELLO, NINO. "Are Left-Handers All Right?" *Mechanics Illustrated,* October, 1969.

LURIA, S.M., MC KAY, CHRISTINE L., and FERRIS, STEVEN H. "Handedness and Adaptation to Visual Distortions of Size and Distance." *Journal of Experimental Psychology,* Vol. 100, No. 2, 1973.

MARTIN, DOUGLAS, and WEBSTER, WILLIAM G. "Paw Preference Shifts in the Rat Following Forced Preference." *Physiology and Behavior,* Vol. 13, December, 1974.

MCKEEVER, WALTER F., VAN DEVENTER, ALLAN D., and SUBERI, MAX. "Avowed, Assessed and Familial Handedness and Differential Hemispheric Processing of Brief Sequential and Non-Sequential Visual Stimuli." *Neuropsychologia,* Vol. 11, May, 1973.

MILLER, EDGAR. "Handedness and the Pattern of Human Ability." *British Journal of Psychology,* Vol. 62, No. 1, 1971.

MILNER, A. D. "Distribution of Hand Preference in Monkeys." *Neuropsychologia,* Vol. 7, May, 1969.

MURRAY, FRANK S., and SAFFERSTONE, JUDITH F. "Pain Threshold and Tolerance of Right and Left Hands." *Journal of Comparative and Physiological Psychology,* Vol. 71, No. 1, 1970.

MYSLOBODSKY, MICHAEL S., and RATTOK, JACK. "Asymmetry of Electrodermal Activity in Man." *Bulletin of the Psychonomic Society,* November, 1975.

NAGYLAKI, THOMAS, and LEVY, JERRE. "The Sound of One Paw Clapping Isn't Sound." *Behavior Genetics,* Vol. 3, No. 3, 1973.

NEBES, ROBERT D. "Handedness and the Perception of Part-Whole Relationship." *Cortex,* December, 1971.

The New Yorker. "The Talk of the Town." May 8, 1971.

NIRENBERG, SUE. "For the Lefty." *House Beautiful,* April, 1974.

ODDY, H. C., and LOBSTEIN, T. J. "Hand and Eye Dominance in Schizophrenia." *British Journal of Psychiatry,* Vol. 120, March, 1972.

OLDFIELD, R . C. "The Assessment and Analysis of Handedness: The Edinburgh Inventory." *Neuropsychologia,* Vol. 9, 1971.

OLSON, GARY M., and LAXAR, KEVIN. "Asymmetries in Processing the Terms 'Right' and 'Left.'" *Journal of Experimental Psychology,* Vol. 100, No. 2, 1973.

PALMER, ROBERT D. "Dimensions of Differentiation in Handedness." *Journal of Clinical Psychology,* October, 1974.

PEARSON, JOHN F. "Making Life Easier for Lefties." *Popular Mechanics,* June, 1971.

PETERSON, GEORGE M., and DEVINE, J. V. "Transfers of Handedness in the Rat Resulting From Small Cortical Lesions After Limited Forced Practice." *Journal of Comparative and Physiological Psychology,* Vol. 56, No. 4, 1963.

PETERSON, JOHN M., and LANSKY, LEONARD M. "Left-Handedness Among Architects: Some Facts and Speculation." *Perceptual and Motor Skills,* Vol. 38, April, 1974.

PFEFFERBAUM, ADOLF, and BUCHSBAUM, MONTE. "Handedness and Cortical Hemisphere Effects in Sine Wave Stimulated Evoked Responses." *Neuropsychologia,* Vol. 9, 1971.

PROVINS, K. A., and CUNLIFFE, PENNY. "The Reliability of Some Motor Performance Tests of Handedness." *Neuropsychologia,* Vol. 10, July, 1972.

Psychology Today. "Southpaws: How Different Are They?" Letter to the Editor. June, 1976.

RACZKOWSKI, DENIS, KALAT, JAMES W., and NEBES, ROBERT. "Reliability and Validity of Some Handedness Questionnaire Items." *Neuropsychologia,* Vol. 12, January, 1974.

SAND, PATRICIA L., and TAYLOR, NEAL. "Handedness: Evaluation of Binomial Distribution Hypothesis in Children and Adults." *Perceptual and Motor Skills,* Vol. 36, June, 1973.

San Francisco Examiner and Chronicle. "The Lefthand Troubles." December 3, 1972.

SATZ, PAUL. "Pathological Left-Handedness: An Explanatory Model." *Cortex,* June, 1972.

SCHREINER, SAMUEL A., JR. "Toward a New Way of Birth." *The Reader's Digest,* January, 1976.

SELIGMANN, JEAN. "Left Hand, Right Hand." *Newsweek,* September 8, 1975.

SPERRY, R. W. "Lateral Specialization of Cerebral Function in the Surgically Separated Hemispheres." *The Psychology of Thinking.* New York: Academic Press, 1973.

STEINGRUEBER, H. J. "Handedness as a Function of Test Complexity." *Perceptual and Motor Skills,* Vol. 40, February, 1975.

Time. "Lefty Liberation." January 7, 1974.

TROTTER, ROBERT J. "Sinister Psychology." *Science News,* October 5, 1974.

TURKEWITZ, GERALD, and CREIGHTON, SUSAN. "Changes in Lateral Differential of Head Posture in the Human Neonate." *Developmental Psychobiology,* Vol. 8, No. 1, 1974.

UHRBROCK, RICHARD S. "Bovine Laterality." *Journal of Genetic Psychology,* Vol. 115, No. 1, 1969.

———. "Laterality in Art." *Journal of Aesthetics and Art Criticism,* Fall, 1973.

VAN BUREN, ABIGAIL. "Dear Abby: Soft in the Heart." *San Francisco Chronicle,* April 8, 1976.

WALKER, HARRY A., and BIRCH, HERBERT G. "Lateral Preference and Right-Left Awareness in Schizophrenic Children." *The Journal of Nervous and Mental Disease,* Vol. 151, No. 5, 1970.

WEBSTER, WILLIAM G., and SHOU, KRISTINE. "Development of Paw Preference in Rats Following Unilateral Cortical Ablations in Infancy." *Perceptual and Motor Skills,* Vol. 40, February, 1975.

WEITEN, WAYNE, and ETAUGH, CLAIRE. "Lateral Eye-Movement Consistency Is Related to Academic Aptitude." *Perceptual and Motor Skills,* Vol. 38, April, 1974.

WIGNER, EUGENE P. "Violations of Symmetry in Physics." *Scientific American,* December, 1965.

WOODWARD, KENNETH L. "When Your Child Can't Read." *McCall's,* February, 1973.

WYATT, RICHARD, and TURSKY, BERNARD. "Skin Potential Levels in Right- and Left-Handed Males." *Psychophysiology,* Vol. 6, No. 2, 1969.

YAKOVLEV, PAUL I. "Motility, Behavior, and the Brain." *The Journal of Nervous and Mental Disease,* April, 1948.

———. "A proposed Definition of the Limbic System." *Limbic System Mechanisms and Autonomic Function.* Charles H. Hockman, Editor. Springfield: Thomas, 1972.

———. "Telokinesis and Handedness: An Empirical Generalization." *Proceedings of the Eighteenth Annual Convention, Society of Biological Psychiatry,* June 7–9, 1973.

——— and RAKIC, PASCO. "Patterns of Decussation of Bulbar Pyramids and Distribution of Pyramidal Tracts on Two Sides of the Spinal Cord." *Transactions of the American Neurological Association,* 1966.

ZIMMERBERG, BETTY, GLICK, STANLEY, and JERUSSI, THOMAS P. "Neurochemical Correlates of a Spatial Preference in Rats." *Science,* August 16, 1974.

Index

211

215